Everyday Gluten-Free

Simple allergen-free cooking with whole foods

by Kim Wilson

See more of the "Everyday Wholesome Eating" series at:
www.simplynaturalhealth.com

Cover design by Linnea Caswell

ISBN 978-0-9831312-0-5

First Printing 2010
Printed in the United States of America

Table of Contents

Cookies, Bars and Brownies

Puddings, Pies and other Desserts

Discussions

A Brief Introduction to

Whole Foods Gluten-free Cooking

How is whole foods gluten-free different?

The ingredients in readily-available gluten-free products and recipes include predominantly refined foods (white rice flour, potato starch, etc.) and starches and gums that are lacking in nutrition and fiber. Not only are these ingredients not beneficial to your health, but they are all fairly unfamiliar, more difficult to come by and more costly than whole natural ingredients.

There are significant health benefits and cost savings to preparing your own whole natural gluten-free foods, but I feel that one of the greatest advantages is that the whole family can partake of the same foods!

Not only gluten-free, but also free of other potentially problematic foods, too!

All the recipes in my books are free of animal products and dairy (which tend to very problematic for people in general) and also free of refined products (flours, sugars, oils, etc.) and common allergens like yeast, soy, and eggs. Many individuals diagnosed with celiac disease and other conditions that require avoiding gluten also find they do best to also avoid dairy, eggs and other allergenic foods. For this reason, I have included dairy-free and egg-free recipes for some common foods (like mayonnaise, sour cream, cheese sauce, ice cream). Corn and oats are two other foods that are sometimes problematic for people, so I include them selectively in recipes

There are a variety of recipes with and without these ingredients. Nuts are another common allergen but can be left out of any recipe without greatly changing it.

1

My hope is that any family needing to eat gluten-free will find within this collection of recipes a repertoire of reliable staples to make gluten-free a doable and healthful lifestyle! That not only will they avoid the problems associated with consuming gluten, but they find their overall health improving with the inclusion of these nutritionally dense foods!

Using gluten-free flours and soaking whole grains
We basically have two options when working with gluten-free ingredients. We can **begin with flour** (either purchased already ground or ground at home- I use a Vitamix with the dry container for this purpose, though there are a lot of great grain mills available also) or we can **presoak the grains**, nuts, seeds or legumes and then blend them together in a recipe. I refer to these recipes as "Blender" recipes.

Soaking ingredients prior to use neutralizes the natural enzyme inhibitors present in seeds/grains. It also begins the germination process, which changes the fats, carbs and sugars in such a way that they even more nutritious and beneficial to our bodies.

Presoaking doesn't take a whole lot of extra time- just some forethought. It actually reduces the amount of work you need to do just prior to cooking. The flavor and texture of baked goods prepared in this way is superior to those made with gluten-free flours and is much more similar to that of the white flour products to which we're accustomed. It is also less costly than using store-bought gluten-free flours.

The advantage of presoaking is great as we both increase the nutritional value and digestibility of the food. This is the ideal way to use whole ingredients as it is more natural and compatible and beneficial to the human body. It isn't always the easiest, however, as it requires some preplanning, so I offer recipes in this book that feature utilize both methods.

Another benefit of "Blender" recipes is that they **freeze well** due to the improved texture from the soaking process.

More than just baked goods

A number of the recipes included in this book wouldn't traditionally contain gluten, yet take into consideration that many people with gluten issues also have other food allergies or sensitivities. For instance, smoothies, sour cream, cheese sauce and ice cream normally contain dairy products, a problem food for many celiacs. Some of the other recipes included are simply great staple recipes- favorites from some of my other cookbooks that help round out a person's diet. If you find yourself in need of more general allergen-free recipes (like soups, salads and entrees) be sure to check out my other recipe books at www.simplynaturalhealth.com.

Why so many pancakes?

I've found that pancakes, biscuits and flatbreads are wonderful alternatives to traditional yeast breads for those on a gluten-free diet. Gluten-free ingredients obviously do not contain the gluten that works in harmony with yeast to produce light, fluffy breads, rolls and other common baked goods.

3

Many attempts are made with refined and less-than-natural ingredients to produce a result similar to that of yeasted wheat breads, but I don't want to sacrifice the quality of my ingredients to achieve a desired effect. I'd rather prepare foods that work well with the inherent characteristics of the natural whole ingredients. Besides tasting great, pancakes, biscuits and flatbreads made from whole natural gluten-free ingredients are significantly more nutritious and beneficial to you than any of the breads you've been accustomed to!

Many may balk at the idea of giving up traditional breads, yet I've come to appreciate that in many cultures and throughout history, people have subsisted on grain-based foods that look a lot more like pancakes, flatbreads and crackers. It's only in more recent history that we have had yeasted breads and bread products and it is predominantly only in Western cultures that we believe it is an essential part of our diet.

My hope is that some of these recipes will encourage individuals to let go of the constant quest for something that is just like "bread" in the gluten-free world. On a day-to-day basis, these other forms of bread can satisfy most needs. You may want to treat yourself occasionally to a prepared gluten-free bread or bread mix, but on a regular basis they really aren't best for our health as they are greatly lacking in nutrition and fiber.

I hope this little collection fills the need for some simple, wholesome gluten-free basics for you!

Setting Up a Gluten-free Pantry

If you've spent any time exploring gluten-free cookbooks or information online, you know there are a million different foods a person with gluten-sensitivity needs to avoid. You've also probably quickly learned that there is quite a list of alternative grains, flours and starches suggested as replacements for the ingredients you're accustomed to. If you've sample many (in prepared foods, mixes or from scratch in recipes), you may be pretty discouraged. Many years ago when I learned I had a wheat allergy I made many of these mixes and recipes and felt I was doomed to eating bean-flavored brownies. Thankfully, in the meantime, I've been encouraged to seek out and experiment with each of the whole foods that are naturally gluten-free. I found many did not appeal (in terms of flavor or texture) and I removed them from my potential "staple ingredients" list. I like to keep things simple, so I was pleased to arrive at six basic gluten-free whole grain flours to work with and also a handful of other gluten-free ingredients that perform well together.

The six flours are: brown rice, sorghum, light buckwheat, teff, oats (certified gluten-free) and cornmeal/corn flour. Two are potential allergens (corn and oat) so they are used selectively in recipes, and alternative ingredients are often offered. Teff may be more difficult to locate, so, likewise, I only use this ingredient occasionally. Brown rice, sorghum and light buckwheat will work best for most people, so they translate into staple ingredients in my recipes.

Keep in stock plenty of the whole grains- brown rice, millet and raw buckwheat groats- as these are excellent soaked and blended in some really basic, really tasty recipes.

In terms of other "staple" components to gluten-free baking, **ground flax** and **apple cider vinegar** are essential. Ground flax combined with water makes a wonderful egg substitute, providing great binding for gluten-free flours that are naturally a bit "crumbly". Keep a pint or more of freshly ground flax in a canning jar on your refrigerator or freezer door so you'll always be prepared to whip up a gluten-free item. Apple cider vinegar enhances the flavor and digestibility of the gluten-free grains and also works with baking powder and baking soda to enhance their leavening effect.

Lastly, you'll notice that many recipes list **"oil/butter"** as an ingredient. I don't specific what kind of oil/butter should be used in each recipe- I leave that up to you. I tend to use coconut butter or oil for baking purposes, and olive oil for preparing dressings, sauces and some stove-top cooking.

Pantry Inventory Guides

The next two pages are handy in providing a basic overview of what I use as my essential gluten-free ingredients. If you stock up on these, you'll be in great shape to prepare almost all of the recipes in this book.

Six Basic Gluten-free Whole Grain Flours

Brown rice flour has a neutral flavor and nice texture. It is a staple ingredient in many recipes. Because it can be gritty if not adequately hydrated, it's beneficial to presoak the brown rice flour with wet ingredients, if time allows.

Sorghum flour has a fairly neutral flavor and yet a finer texture than brown rice flour. It combines especially well with corn, naturally complementing the corn flavor.

Light buckwheat flour has a slight distinct flavor but is highly nutritious and adds nice texture, so it is great to add a small portion to most recipes.

Teff has great texture, but because it has a distinct flavor (pleasant, yet only suitable for certain applications) and has limited availability, it is only included selectively in recipes.

Certified gluten-free oats contribute "warmth", sweetness, and heartiness plus good nutrition to baked goods. Some people have difficulty with even GF oats, so I use it selectively.

Cornmeal/Corn flour adds nice flavor and texture to baked goods. We especially like it in breads that will be toasted as well as added to pizza crust. Again, some people have sensitivities to this ingredient, however, so it is only included occasionally.

Whole Grains for Gluten-free Baking

Brown rice (medium to long grain for "blender" recipes)
Raw hulled buckwheat groats
Millet
GF rolled oats or steel-cut oats

Enhancers for Gluten-free Baking

Raw apple cider vinegar
Flax seed (ground and mixed with water as a binding agent,
        much like eggs)
Nut meal (almond, hazelnut, pecan) - only used occasionally,
        in small portions, to provide richness to a recipe
Leavening- baking powder, baking soda, apple cider vinegar
Fat/oils- olive oil, coconut oil/butter, organic butter
Sweeteners- honey, agave syrup, maple syrup, molasses

Other Staples for Gluten-free Cooking

Whole grains - *for use in side dishes, cereals, entrees, etc.*
brown rice, raw hulled buckwheat groats, buckwheat kasha,
cornmeal (grits, polenta), millet, quinoa, certified gluten-free
rolled oats and steel-cut oats
Beans/legumes- *in whole or flour form-primarily for making
bean/lentil cakes (as a bread/pita substitute)*
lentils, chana dal, gram flour, etc.

Information on
Specific Ingredients

Gluten-free Oats

Oats are a wonderful addition to baked goods. They contribute heartiness, a nice texture and mild, sweet flavor. They bind well and are dense and moist, but can seem a bit too "pasty" if used in too great a proportion. Oats are full of great fiber, nutrition and healthy fats (especially beneficial for young people). Enough people avoid oats (because of the gluten content due to cross-contamination in standard oats, the expense of certified gluten-free oats and/or other problems with oats) that I include oats selectively in my recipes. For instance, my "Oatmeal Chocolate Chip Cake" (page 88) just wouldn't be right without oats! Rarely are oats a main ingredient (for a delicious exception, try the "Oat Biscuit" recipe, page 56) yet many of the recipes in my first wheat-free baking book featured oats and light buckwheat as the key ingredients. Many of the recipes that include oats offer a possible substitution for those who don't do well with them.

You can easily grind oat flour in a blender from certified gluten-free rolled oats or steel-cut oats:

2 cups of rolled oat equals about 2 cups ground oat flour
2 cups of steel-cut oats equals about 2 ¾ cups oat flour

Buckwheat and Its Many Varieties

Buckwheat is an interesting ingredient. Technically it is not a grain, but the seed of an herb, so very few people have any digestive or health issues related to consuming it. Many are often confused by its name, however, assuming that it is in the wheat family. It is no relation and you can be assured that it is gluten-free. Most people are familiar with buckwheat pancakes, made from traditional buckwheat flour which is naturally gray in color. It is the only form of buckwheat that I don't use regularly. It is made from the buckwheat groat with the dark hull intact (hence the color) and has a stronger flavor than what I refer to as "light buckwheat flour". I haven't found it a pleasant addition or key ingredient to any gluten-free recipes except for "Buckwheat Pancakes", page 28. More commonly I use whole raw hulled buckwheat groats and the flour ground from such in my recipes.

Buckwheat is packed with an abundance of nutrition. It is a superb source of high quality protein, minerals, fiber and even antioxidants. For this reason, it is beneficial to add some light buckwheat flour (the flour ground from raw hulled buckwheat groats) to gluten-free recipes in order to boost the nutritional content.

Raw/hulled buckwheat groats- hulled whole buckwheat
> Great in cereals and ground into flour

Kasha- toasted buckwheat groats, makes tasty side dishes

Traditional buckwheat flour- gray in color, earthy flavor
> Good in traditional buckwheat pancakes

Light/raw buckwheat flour (ground hulled buckwheat)
> Great addition to gluten-free recipes

Light Buckwheat Flour

When I use buckwheat flour in a recipe, I am using what I refer to as "raw" or "light" buckwheat flour. This is flour ground from the whole raw buckwheat kernel, but without the dark hull. When you purchase whole raw hulled buckwheat and grind it into flour, you get much lighter colored and flavored flour and this is great added to many recipes. It has a distinct flavor that can come across too strong if used in too great a proportion, but it contributes some great nutrition, binding and texture, so is a beneficial addition to many gluten-free recipes. The inclusion of apple cider vinegar helps mellow this.

It can easily be ground into flour in a blender.

2 cups of raw buckwheat groats equals about 2 ¾ cups flour

Cornmeal/Corn Flour

Try to find stoneground, wholegrain cornmeal (not degerminated). Blue cornmeal contains even greater amounts of minerals than yellow and is usually less problematic for those who find they have a sensitivity to corn. I've found that corn and buckwheat are not complementary but corn and sorghum, on the other hand, work very well together.

Sorghum Flour

For those who are unfamiliar with sorghum, it is a plant similar to millet. In fact, when I've purchased sorghum flour at an Indian grocery (called "jowar flour" there) the English description reads "white millet flour".

Teff Flour

Teff is an African grain, traditionally used to make injera (a large flatbread) in Ethiopia. Teff has a distinct flavor that works well with bananas, chocolate and spices. Nutritionally, it has more protein than wheat and has a far superior portion of iron, calcium and other minerals.

Beans and Bean Flours

I was pleasantly surprised to find that pancakes made from some varieties of soaked beans and legume flours have a more pleasant texture and flavor than some gluten-free grains. This is a great discovery because the nutrition and fiber found in beans make a wonderful contribution to our diet and health.

Chana dal or Gram/Besan Flour- Chana dal is described as a split chick pea, but it is quite different from what we commonly think of as a chick pea. It is an Indian variety that is smaller, rounder and more deeply colored. When chana dal is ground it is called "gram flour" or "besan flour". In both forms, this ingredient has a milder flavor and texture than traditional chickpeas. It has a nice eggy, almost buttery flavor, a fluffy texture and holds together very well.

Many gluten-free recipes feature "chickpea flour" which is ground from the larger, lighter-colored chickpeas we're more familiar with. Traditional chickpeas make great dishes and hummus, but for baking purposes I've found "chickpea flour" quite disappointing. I encourage you to seek out some chana dal or gram/besan flour for your gluten-free cooking. You'll find them in a large health food store or coop, or at an Indian grocery.

Lentils (soaked and pureed with water) have a nice mild, slightly beany flavor and nice texture. They're particularly good in lentil cakes- a great bread alternative to serve with soup or salad (pg. 32).

Ground Flax

Flax seed is rich in good oils and fiber, yet its oil is highly susceptible to spoilage with exposure to light, heat and air. The oils are protected for as long as the seed is intact; however, we get very little benefit from the seed if we eat it whole. It's important, therefore, to grind flax before using it. It is most healthful and economical to purchase whole flax seeds (brown or golden) and grind them yourself. You can grind them in a coffee grinder or a blender, being careful to not overgrind as this overheats the oils. You'll notice that the smell will change if you overgrind or overheat the flax. I shake the coffee grinder while grinding flax and make sure it keeps circulating in the blender in order to minimize the chances of this happening. I find it handy to keep a glass pint or quart **jar of preground flax in the freezer** as this protects the oils from expiring and allows me to avoid grinding fresh flax for each recipe.

Ground flax mixed with water has an "eggy" consistency that helps to bind ingredients together, but also contributes beneficial oils and fiber to baked goods. The flavor is very mild, slightly nutty, so does not detract from the overall flavor of baked goods. You can mix **1 Tbsp. of ground flax with 3 Tbsp. water as the replacement for one egg**.

Ground flax can also be **sprinkled** on hot or cold cereal or on top of fruit smoothies or salad. It can also be used as a **supplement**- just mix about 2 Tbsp. with 8 oz. water, followed by another 8 oz. glass of water. This is another great way to benefit from the oils and fiber of ground flax.

Apple Cider Vinegar

You'll notice that grains for "blender" recipes are often soaked overnight in water and vinegar. Vinegar is also added to many baked good recipes. This may seem odd at first exposure, yet the inclusion of vinegar in these recipes is quite intentional. The use of an acid (like vinegar) in a grain-based recipe helps to neutralize enzyme inhibitors and anti-nutrients naturally present in the grains. It also improves the texture of the finished product as it reacts with baking powder and baking soda, creating a leavening effect similar to that of eggs. If you used non-dairy milk in a baked good recipe as a substitute for water, add 1-2 tsp. of apple cider vinegar to it in advance of adding to the recipe. It will contribute a sour milk effect- a richer finished product, especially with pancakes.

Raw buckwheat makes a great contribution to recipes (nutritionally and texture-wise) but sometimes the flavor comes through too strongly. The inclusion of apple cider vinegar in a recipe with this flour tends to mellow the flavor.

I specify raw apple cider vinegar because it is the most healthful variety of vinegars. White vinegar should be reserved for cleaning purposes in the home.

Recommended Kitchen Tools

"Got to have" items for a serious gluten-free cook are a heavy-duty blender and at least one good cast iron skillet.

A **heavy-duty blender** is essential for grinding all kinds of grains and blending all kinds of batters. We also use ours daily for making fruit smoothies, salad dressings and such.

At the present time we have four nicely-seasoned **cast iron skillets**. I don't think I've ever purchased one new. They must have been thrift-store finds or passed down to me. I love our really shallow skillet for making pancakes. To keep your skillet in good condition be sure to never wash it. No water. No soap. Just wipe it out with a paper towel after using. If it is quite dry, add a little oil before wiping it out.

I also really like **baking stones** and **ceramic or glass baking dishes**. When making cakes and muffins I often don't bother oiling the baking dishes. I find that after a short soak in the sink the pans clean up easily enough. As an added bonus, the dishes used for gluten-free baked goods clean up more easily than those used for baking with traditional ingredients.

If you don't have a baking stone, by all means, treat yourself to some **baking parchment paper**. This makes baking clean-up a breeze! I resisted baking for years because I dreaded washing the baking sheets. Little did I know that ordeal could have been avoided with the use of parchment paper!

Quite a number of my recipes are called "Blender" recipes because they are prepared in a blender from soaked grains. These recipes are great tasting and great for you. A **fine mesh strainer** is a handy tool for these "blender" recipes as the soaked grains will fall through a traditional sieve.

And a couple last "luxury items" (though they aren't that costly) are a **push-up measuring cup** (great for measuring coconut butter, nut butters, honey, etc.) and an **ice cream scoop** (great for portioning muffin and biscuit batter).

Working With Gluten-free Ingredients and Recipes

Variations in amounts in recipes: You'll notice that I sometimes include options in amounts of certain ingredients in recipes. I often give a range with sweeteners because some people want to use the minimal amount and other people want it to taste as similar as possible to a traditional baked good. Sometimes options are given for salt and spices as well, also allowing for individual taste.

Flour Substitutions: When working with gluten-free flours you have some flexibility in substituting one flour for another. Because of the differences in fineness of the flours, however, it isn't always a one-to-one substitution. Play around with the recipes to find a density and texture that is pleasing to you.

When brown rice flour is substituted for another flour, about ¼ more water/liquid needs to be added for proper hydration.

Because oat flour is so fine, you'll need to use about half again as much in recipes when substituting for another flour.

Sorghum flour, teff flour and light buckwheat flour are pretty much interchangeable in terms of their texture (though the flavor will change, so you'll want to experiment with this).

Please remember every recipe in this book
was created through trial-and-error.
You have the same ability through experimentation
to come up with even greater recipes!

Batter appears too thin
Because gluten-free flours tend to be coarser than wheat flour, they require more liquids to become properly hydrated. Because of this, the batter for cakes, muffins and other baked goods may initially appear too thin. Don't worry. The final product will be great!

Let baked goods "rest"
Gluten free baked goods will seem too gummy if you attempt to slice and serve them directly out of the oven. They benefit from a "rest"- an amount of time to cool a bit before being handled. I can't explain why this is exactly, but I suspect it is similar to how rice shouldn't be stirred soon after cooking, but also benefits from a rest in the pot for the moisture to settle.

Allow time for flours to adequately hydrate
Gluten-free flours tend to be coarser than traditional wheat flour, so they require more liquids and more "hydration" time. If you have the time, it's a good idea to combine most of the flours (reserve a little bit to mix the baking powder or baking soda into before adding just before cooking) with the liquids. A "sit" time before baking (from minutes to hours) will improve the texture of the final product.

Ground flax combined with wet ingredients
In most recipes the ground flax should be mixed with the wet ingredients prior to combining with dry ingredients. The ground flax then has an opportunity to absorb water and become an eggy consistency that works well in binding the gluten-free ingredients together. An exception to this is in the baking mixes, where the ground flax is combined with the dry ingredients. Extra flax is added to these blends for that reason.

Want a cake or other baked good to be moister?
Adding more water, applesauce and/or oil/butter will increase the moistness of a baked good. Adding more ground flax also serves to hold the moistness for a greater length of time.

For thickening purposes: Brown rice flour thickens well (but not as smooth as other flours), oat flour produces a nice smooth consistency (a bit "gummy" when a lot of flour is used- good for applications like cheese sauce) and sorghum flour is a good smooth thickener with a neutral flavor.

Gluten-free Breakfast Options

Fresh fruit

Fruit salad

Fruit smoothie

Trail mix/Snack mix

Muesli

Buckwheat Fruit and Nut Cereal

Hot GF cereal (like baked oatmeal or cream of rice)

Pancakes

Waffles

Muffins

Bread with
    butter, nutbutter,
    jelly, honey, etc.

Wholesome Snack Ideas

Fresh fruit

Dried fruit

Fruit salad

Fruit smoothie

Applesauce

Snack/trail mix

Nut-stuffed dates

Nut butter on celery,
    apples, bananas

Cut veggies and dip

Nuts (almonds, pecans,
    walnuts, etc.)

Seeds (pumpkin,
    sunflower, etc.)

GF muffins

GF cookies/bars

GF bread/toast

GF cake

GF crackers

GF chips

Tortilla chips with
    salsa or guacamole

Hummus with chips
    or cut veggies

Popcorn

Muesli

GF cereal

GF hot cereal

GF oatmeal

Gluten-free Lunch Options

Soup with: pancakes, waffles, lentil cakes, chana dal cakes,
    bread, cornbread, flatbread, corn muffins,
    biscuits, crackers, tortilla chips, etc.

Pocket sandwich- split open a lentil or chana dal cake
    and stuff with salad, grilled veggies, etc.

Nutbutter and jelly sandwich on:
    sliced, plain or toasted basic bread or blender bread
    chana dal cake/waffle

Hummus with cut veggies and GF chips, crackers or
    flatbread

GF tortilla chips or crackers with refried beans, salsa,
    guacamole, etc.

Beans and rice- served with fresh chopped tomatoes,
    lettuce, and onions plus salsa, guacamole,
    sunflower sour cream, cheese sauce, etc.

Bean burritos/soft tacos- made with corn or GF tortillas

Leftover chili with tortilla chips

Baked potatoes with toppings- grilled veggies, broccoli,
    sunflower sour cream, cheese sauce, etc.

GF pasta with pasta sauce

Salad with lots of toppings (veggies, nuts, seeds, beans,
    dried fruit, etc.,) and served with crackers, flatbread,
    lentil cakes, etc.

Muesli or Buckwheat Fruit and Nut Cereal
    with nut milk or banana milk

Hot GF cereal (baked oatmeal, cream of rice, etc.)

Pancakes or waffles

Traveling Gluten-free

Pack plenty of snacks (lots of fresh fruit, dried fruit, nuts, trail mix, homemade or prepared GF snacks)

Bring along tried-and-true prepared GF foods that you may not be able to locate (bread, pasta, chips, crackers, etc.)

GF bread, nutbutter and jelly for on the road (even gluten-free pancakes work well for this purpose)

GF chips- rice, corn, potato, legume-based

Popcorn

Eating Out Gluten-free

Investigate restaurants that might be a good option
Many restaurants now offer gluten-free information online and more and more restaurants offer gluten-free options.

Steak houses- often have a good salad bar, baked potatoes and great "veggie of the day" selections

Ethnic Restaurants- often offer great gluten-free entrees

    Chinese   Korean   Mexican

    Indian   Thai

Worst case scenario- (at common franchise restaurants)

    Put together a meal from the "sides" menu:

        Side salad (some have salad bars)

        Roast or baked potatoes

        Steamed, grilled veggies

Surviving the Holidays and Special Occasions Gluten-free

Call ahead to get an understanding of what will be available
Prepare a bread/pasta alternative for those who need it
Offer to bring something. Some easy, well-received options:

Large salad with toppings and dressings
Hummus with cut veggies and tortilla chips
Tortilla chips with salsa and/or guacamole
Chili with cornbread, brown rice, or tortilla chips
A platter of Nut-stuffed Dates or Fruit and Nut Balls
Blueberry cobbler
Apple crisp

Especially for the Kids

Parties- eat ahead of time, enjoying some special foods or treats so you/your children feel less deprived at the party or bring along alternatives/substitutions (cake, ice cream, etc.).

Allergenic "treats"- Keep a "stash" of allergen-free treats at home and/or in your car so your children will be able to "trade up" when they've been given problematic foods by others.

Hurray for Pancakes!

As I began experimenting with recipes, I became impressed by what an easy and satisfying option gluten-free pancakes are. I almost want to call them something else, like "skillet cakes", because I want to disassociate them from their "breakfast-only" reputation. I've also found that whipping up a batch of simple gluten-free "cakes" (pancakes or skillet cakes) doesn't take much longer than it did to toast some bread to serve with a meal. I just don't get to walk away from the stovetop as I could with a toaster.

Pancakes are great on their own, but can also be used like bread as well. Spread with butter, nut butter or jelly or serve with soup or salad. They make a really quick and easy breakfast for the kids too. Just mix up some batter with a little gluten-free flour, water, salt and oil, cook a couple of minutes on a skillet and -voila- tasty cakes ready for consumption!

I have a few bread recipes in this book, yet offer many more options for pancakes, biscuits and flatbreads because I find these a handier and quicker alternative to traditional yeast breads.

Basic Pancakes/Waffles

1 cup corn flour*
1 cup GF oat flour
½ cup brown rice flour
2 tsp. baking powder
½ tsp. sea salt

2 cups non-dairy milk**
2 tsp. apple cider vinegar
3 Tbsp. ground flax
2 Tbsp. oil/butter
1-2 Tbsp. honey

PANCAKES: Mix dry ingredients (left column) in a large mixing bowl. Add vinegar to the non-dairy milk and allow to "sour" for a couple of minutes (You can skip this step and/or use water in place of the milk). Combine wet ingredients in right column (including "soured milk"). Lightly mix wet into dry ingredients. Add a bit more water if the batter seems too thick. Cook on a hot oiled griddle till cakes are browned on each side. **Makes about 2 dozen 3 ½ inch pancakes**

* or fine cornmeal
**or water

WAFFLES: Add another tablespoon or two of oil to the batter before cooking in a hot waffle iron.

Pancake and Waffle Toppings

Butter, coconut butter, flax oil
Raw honey, maple syrup, agave
Chopped strawberries, berry sauce
Sautéed bananas (in butter and maple syrup)
Applesauce

Cornmeal Pancakes

1 cup cornmeal*
1 1/2 cup GF oat flour
1 tsp. sea salt
2 tsp. baking powder

2 cups water
2 Tbsp. ground flax
2 Tbsp. oil/butter
1 tsp. apple cider vinegar
opt: 1-2 Tbsp. honey

Separately mix ingredients in two columns (dry and wet). Combine and then allow to set for at least 5-10 minutes before cooking. Cook on hot oiled skillet until bubbles form on surface. Flip and cook till lightly browned.

This batter also comes out great when allowed to set for several hours (even overnight in the refrigerator) before cooking. Add a little more water if the batter is too thick when ready to prepare.

Makes about 2 dozen 3 ½ inch pancakes

* wholegrain blue or yellow cornmeal

Teff Pancakes

2 ½ cups teff flour
2 tsp. baking powder
½ tsp. sea salt

2 cups water
2 Tbsp. oil/butter
1 Tbsp. ground flax
2 tsp. apple cider vinegar

Mix dry ingredients (left column) in a bowl. Combine ingredients in right column then add to dry, mixing lightly. Cook on a medium skillet, until lightly browned on each side.
Makes about 2 dozen 3 ½ inch pancakes

Pancake Variations:

Blueberry pancakes: add ¾ cup blueberries to batter.

To make waffles- reduce amount of water slightly and add an additional 1-2 Tbsp. of oil/butter to batter.

Pancake Syrup

Whisk together 2 parts maple syrup and 1 part flax oil. Drizzle over pancakes or waffles.

Banana Teff Pancakes

1 ½ cup water
1- 1 ½ bananas
2 Tbsp. oil/butter
1 tsp. apple cider vinegar

1 ¼ cup teff flour
2/3 cup brown rice flour*
2 tsp. baking powder
1/4-1/2 tsp. sea salt

Combine wet ingredients (left column). Process them in a blender to get the banana nice and smooth or just hand mash the banana before combining with the other ingredients. Mix dry ingredients (right column) and then combine with the wet. Cook on a medium-low skillet for a couple of minutes on each side. **Makes about 2 dozen 3 ½ inch pancakes**
* or 1 cup GF oat flour

Variation: replace bananas with ½- 3/4 cup applesauce and add ½ tsp. cinnamon for apple cinnamon pancakes.

These are great topped with butter and/or maple syrup!

Buckwheat Pancakes

2 cups buckwheat flour*   2 1/2 cups water
¾ cup brown rice flour   2 Tbsp. oil/butter
2 tsp. baking powder   2 Tbsp. ground flax
1/2 + tsp. sea salt   2 tsp. apple cider vinegar

Separately mix ingredients in two columns (dry and wet). Combine. Allow to rest for a couple of minutes. Cook on hot skillet until bubbles form. Flip and cook on other side until lightly browned.

Makes about 2 dozen 3 ½ inch pancakes

*This is the one instance in this book where traditional gray-colored buckwheat flour is used. It makes heavy, earthy-flavored pancakes. You can presift the buckwheat flour for improved texture.

Lazy Mixing Method

Instead of using two separate bowls when mixing up pancakes or baked goods, I often just add the flours on top of the already combined wet ingredients and then lightly mix the baking powder and sea salt into the top of the flour pile before whisking it all together.

Blender Pancakes/Waffles

1 1/4 cup brown rice

3/4 cup whole millet*

Opt: 2-3 Tbsp. sesame seeds

2 Tbsp. apple cider vinegar

_____

2 tsp. baking powder

1 3/4 - 2 cups water

2 Tbsp. oil/butter

1 Tbsp. honey**

1 tsp. apple cider vinegar

2 Tbsp. ground flax

3/4- 1 tsp. sea salt

Soak brown rice and millet (and sesame seeds) in a bowl with water and vinegar for at least 8 hours (overnight works well). Drain the grains (and seeds) and then add to a blender with the rest of the ingredients, except for baking powder. Process until smooth. Add baking powder and blend briefly. Pour batter onto a medium hot skillet and cook for a couple of minutes on each side.

*or raw hulled buckwheat

** or agave or maple syrup

Makes over 3 dozen 3 ½ inch pancakes

Variation: replace 1/4 cup of the water with a ripe banana or cored apple

For waffles: add an additional tablespoon or oil/butter and pour batter into a hot waffle iron.

Blender pancakes are my favorites not just because of their exceptional flavor and texture (they're light like more traditional white flour pancakes), but also for their nutritional value. I love them because you begin with whole grains which you soak overnight (beginning the germination process- which increases nutrition and digestibility, and the soaking process also gets rid of any anti-nutrients naturally present in grains- like phytates). Then it is super easy the next day to drain the grains, add with water and other ingredients to a blender and whip them up. And what could be handier than the convenience of pouring the batter directly from the blender container onto the skillet?! The optional sesame seeds add extra nutritional value- particularly calcium.

Blender Recipes

You'll find a number of "blender" recipes in this book. This means whole grains were soaked for a period of time to allow for the breakdown of enzyme inhibitors and to increase nutritional value, and then are processed in blender for use in a pancake, muffin, cake or cookie recipe. The texture of baked goods made from blended soaked grains is superior to those made with gluten-free flours and is much more similar to that of the white flour products we're accustomed to. They are more nutritious and more economical to make too! "Blender" recipes are my favorites and definitely worth the effort to set some grains to soak ahead of time.

Chana Dal Cakes/Waffles

2 cups chana dal
2 Tbsp. oil/butter

2 ½ cups water
1 tsp. sea salt

Presoak beans for at least four hours (ideally overnight).

Drain beans and then blend with the rest of the ingredients until smooth. Cook for a few minutes on each side on a medium-low skillet.
For waffles: Cook batter in a hot waffle iron.

*These pancakes are very tasty
and go great with soup or salad.
We like to slice them open like a pita and
stuff with salad and dressing. Easy and yummy.*

Chana dal *is the Indian name for split desi chickpeas. They are smaller than traditional chickpeas. You can get them at many health food stores as well as Indian grocery stores.*

Variation: Moong dal or urid dal can be substituted for the chana dal. The flavors are slightly different (moong dal more "beany" and urid dal quite mild).

Lentil Cakes

Presoak for at least 2 hours:

> 1 cup lentils, split peas or split mung beans

3/4 cup water	1/2 tsp. ground cumin
1/2 onion	1/4 tsp. turmeric
2 cloves garlic	pinch cinnamon
3/4 tsp. sea salt	pinch cayenne
opt: 1/2 tsp. ground ginger	1 Tbsp. parsley (later)
opt: 4 sliced scallions	

Puree all ingredients, except for lentils and parsley, in food processor or blender. Drain lentils and add to mixture, pureeing till smooth. Mix in parsley (and scallions). Drop onto an oiled skillet, cooking a few minutes per side.
Variation: leave out spices for a more neutral flavor.

These cakes are even better when reheated.
The texture and flavor gets even better over time.

*You might be tempted to pass this recipe by, but I encourage you to **give it a try**. These little cakes have become staples for many families! They make tasty soup or salad accompaniments and can be cut open like a pita and stuffed with salad and dressing or grilled vegetables. Yum!*

Basic Muffin Recipe

2 cups GF flour (see below)

2 tsp. baking powder

½ tsp. sea salt

up to 1 1/2 tsp. spice

2/3 -1 cup additions

    -nuts, raisins, fruit, chips, etc.

1 cup water*

1/2 cup applesauce

1/3 cup sweetener**

1/4 cup oil/butter

1 tsp. apple cider vinegar

1/3 cup ground flax

Combine wet ingredients (right column) in a mixing bowl. Either mix dry ingredients in a separate bowl and then combine with wet ingredients or use my " "lazy-man's method" that eliminates the need for a second mixing bowl—measure dry ingredients on top of the wet mixture and gently stir the baking powder and salt into the flour before combining with the wet ingredients. Scoop into oiled muffin cups (an ice cream scoop works great for this). Bake at 400 degrees for 18-20 minutes. ***Makes one dozen muffins***

* or non-dairy milk

** honey, agave or maple syrup

Flour Options

Any of the flour blends used in the baking mixes work great for making muffins. You can also make simpler combinations like:

      brown rice (1 ¼ cup) and teff or sorghum (3/4 cup),

      sorghum (1 ¼ cup) and corn or teff (3/4 cup), etc.

Muffin Variations

Date nut- dates, pecans, cinnamon

Maple walnut- maple syrup, walnuts

Cinnamon apple- applesauce, cinnamon, chopped apple

Carrot raisin- cinnamon, ginger, shredded carrot, raisins

Lemon poppy- honey, lemon juice and zest, poppy seeds

Chocolate chip- chocolate (or carob) chips, nuts, cinnamon

Pineapple coconut- crushed pineapple and juice, coconut

"Surprise" muffins- pour muffin cups half full with batter, add 1 Tbsp. all-fruit jelly, then finish filling cup with batter.

*For nice light muffins, mix batter as briefly
as possible before scooping into muffin cups.*

Streusel Topping

1/2 cup sorghum flour*
1 tsp. cinnamon
pinch of sea salt

3 Tbsp. maple syrup
1 ½ Tbsp. oil/butter

With a fork, combine streusel topping ingredients, then crumble or drizzle over muffins or cake before baking.
* or ½ cup light buckwheat flour or 2/3 cup oat flour

Cinnamon Raisin Muffins

1 cup brown rice flour
2/3 cup sorghum flour
1/3 cup light buckwheat flour
2 tsp. baking powder
1 1/2 tsp. cinnamon
½ tsp. sea salt
1 cup raisins

1 cup water
1/4 cup oil/butter
1/3 cup honey*
1/2 cup applesauce
1 tsp. apple cider vinegar
1/3 cup ground flax
opt: ¾ cup chopped nuts

Combine wet ingredients (right column) in a mixing bowl. Combine dry ingredients and then mix with wet ingredients. Scoop into oiled muffin cups. Bake at 400 degrees for 18-20 minutes. **_Makes one dozen muffins_**
* or agave or maple syrup

*This is an example of use of the Basic Baking Mix flour blend.
This recipe also works well with the
Oat Buckwheat Baking Mix flour blend.*

Banana Walnut Muffins

3-4 bananas, mashed

1/2 cup water

¼ cup oil/butter

1/3 cup honey

1 tsp. apple cider vinegar

1/3 cup ground flax

¾-1 cup chopped walnuts

1 cup brown rice flour

2/3 cup teff flour*

1/3 cup light buckwheat flour

2 tsp. baking powder

½ tsp. baking soda

½ tsp. sea salt

1 tsp. cinnamon

Combine wet ingredients (left column except for walnuts). In a separate bowl combine dry ingredients (right column). Lightly mix the two together and then fold in the walnuts. Scoop into oiled muffin cups. Bake at 400 degrees for about 20 minutes.   ***Makes one dozen muffins***

* or sorghum flour

Cranberry Nut Muffins

1 1/3 cup GF oat flour

1/3 cup brown rice flour

1/3 cup light buckwheat flour*

½ tsp. cinnamon

2 tsp. baking powder

½ tsp. sea salt

3/4 cup chopped nuts

1 cup orange juice
    or pineapple juice

½ cup honey**

3 Tbsp. oil/butter

½ cup ground flax

1 cup cranberries

opt: 1 Tbsp. orange zest

Combine dry ingredients (left column) in a large mixing bowl. Lightly chop cranberries. Combine the ingredients in the right column (except for cranberries) and then mix with the dry ingredients (and zest, if using). Fold in cranberries. Scoop into muffins cups and bake at 400 degrees for 25-30 minutes.

Makes one dozen muffins

* or sorghum flour

** or agave or maple syrup

Double Chocolate Muffins

1 1/3 cup warm water
¼ cup oil/butter
½ cup honey*
1/2 cup applesauce**
2 tsp. apple cider vinegar
1/3 cup ground flax

1 cup brown rice flour
3/4 cup teff flour***
1/3 cup cocoa powder
2 tsp. baking powder
1/2 tsp. sea salt
1/2 cup chocolate chips
opt: 1/3 cup chopped walnuts

Combine ingredients in left column together. In a large bowl, combine the ingredients on the right (except for chocolate chips (and walnuts, if using). Combine the wet and dry mixtures briefly, then gently mix in chocolate chips (and nuts). Scoop into muffin cups and bake at 400 degrees for about 20 minutes. **Makes one dozen muffins**

*or agave or maple syrup
** or prune puree
*** or ½ cup sorghum flour plus ¼ cup light buckwheat flour

Carob version: replace cocoa powder with carob powder, chocolate chips with carob chips and add 1 tablespoon of molasses and 2 Tbsp. of tahini to batter.

Corn Muffins

1 1/3 cup cornmeal
2/3 cup sorghum flour
2 tsp. baking powder
1/2+ tsp. sea salt

1 1/4 cup warm water
3 Tbsp. honey
3 Tbsp. oil/butter
1 tsp. apple cider vinegar
1/3 cup ground flax

Mix dry ingredients (left column) in a bowl. Combine wet ingredients (right column)- sometimes I just shake them together in a sealed pint jar. Combine wet and dry and scoop into oiled muffin cups (an ice cream scoop works great for this purpose). Bake at 400 degrees for 18-20 minutes.
Makes almost one dozen muffins

Cornmeal and sorghum flour have proved to be a winning combination- their flavors and textures combine well.

Super Good Muffins

3/4 cup GF rolled oats
2/3 cup raisins
2 Tbsp. oil/butter
1 ¼ cup boiling water
1/2 cup applesauce
1/4 cup honey*
3 Tbsp. molasses
2 tsp. apple cider vinegar
1/2 cup ground flax

2/3 cup light buckwheat flour**
2/3 cup sorghum flour**
2 tsp. cinnamon
2 tsp. baking powder
½ tsp. sea salt
opt: 3/4 cup chopped nuts

Pour boiling water over oats, raisins and oil/butter in a small mixing bowl. Whisk in the rest of the ingredients in the left column. Mix dry ingredients in another bowl. Combine the wet and dry ingredients together and scoop into oiled muffin cups. Bake at 400 degrees for 20-24 minutes.

Makes one dozen muffins

* or agave or maple syrup
** or substitute teff flour for either of these flours

These muffins are nutritional powerhouses, with minimal sweeteners and fat. Each muffin has almost 6 grams of fiber, plus over 8% of the iron and almost 5% of the recommended calcium for the day! They also taste great. Originally I named them "Super Yummy Super Good for You Muffins", but that was a little long, so I reduced it to "Super Good".

Banana Blender Muffins

1 1/3 cups brown rice
1/2 cup millet
1/3 cup raw buckwheat
1 Tbsp. apple cider vinegar

_____

2 tsp. baking powder
½ tsp. baking soda

1 1/4 cups water
2-3 ripe bananas
2 Tbsp. oil/butter
3+ Tbsp. honey*
1 tsp. apple cider vinegar
1/4 cup ground flax
1 tsp. cinnamon
¼ tsp. nutmeg
3/4 tsp. sea salt

Soak grains (and sesame seeds) overnight (or for at least 8 hours). Drain and then add to blender with the ingredients in the right column. When batter is quite smooth, gently blend in baking powder and soda (sift through a sieve and whisk in to avoid lumps). Pour into oiled muffin cups. Bake at 400 degrees for about 20 minutes.

Makes more than one dozen muffins

* or agave or maple syrup

Option: add 1 cup of raisins to muffin batter before baking.

*Be sure to oil your muffin cups well so they release easily.
I prefer using a baking stone (muffin top style)
as the clean-up is simplified.*

Fruit Smoothie

2 oranges
2 handfuls of blueberries,
   strawberries, pineapple,
   grapes or whatever fruit
   you may have on hand
   (fresh or frozen)

1/3 cup nuts*
½ cup water or ice
2 frozen bananas
opt: 1 apple (cored)
opt: 2 Tbsp. flax oil

Peel, cut and add fruits to the blender. Add rest of ingredients and puree until smooth. *(I like to puree the orange sections, nuts, water and any 'seedy' berries before adding the other ingredients, to make sure they are thoroughly processed.)*
Variation: In place of the 2 whole oranges, substitute one cup of orange juice (ideally, fresh squeezed).
* walnuts, almonds, pecans, etc.- ideally presoaked overnight.
Fresh bananas instead of frozen? Add some ice in place of some of the water for a better consistency.

Great served topped with chopped nuts (almonds, walnuts, pecans), shredded coconut and/or ground flax.
Try one for breakfast or lunch, or as a snack!

Green Smoothie: add a couple handfuls of spinach
or a few leaves of kale to the blender in final processing. The color and nutritional value will change, but the flavor, remarkably, doesn't change much. A great nutritional boost!

Muesli

8 cups GF rolled oats

1 cup shredded coconut

1 cup sunflower seeds

1/2 cup pumpkin seeds

1 cup chopped nuts

2 tsp. cinnamon

1 1/2 cup raisins

1/2 cup chopped dried fruit

(apricots, prunes, figs, dates)

opt: 1/2 cup ground flax*

Combine ingredients then store in the refrigerator or freezer.

Makes 12 cups

* Ideally, add freshly ground flax at time of serving.

Muesli can be enjoyed:

plain (as a snack),

in a bowl topped with banana or nut milk (as cereal),

or presoaked overnight (equal parts muesli and water)

and mixed with mashed banana when ready to serve.

It's also great topped with some chopped fresh fruit!

Buckwheat Fruit and Nut Cereal

¼ cup raw buckwheat groats
¼- ½ cup dried fruits (raisins, dates, figs, apricots, etc.)
¼ - ½ cup nuts, seeds (almonds, pecans, walnuts, etc.)

Cover these ingredients with water and allow to soak at least overnight (8-12 hours). When ready to eat, mix with a mashed banana or banana milk. You can also sprinkle with cinnamon, coconut, ground flax, fresh fruit or applesauce or drizzle with a bit of honey, if desired.

Unless you like a very thick cereal, you'll want to soak the buckwheat separate from the fruits and nuts. Thoroughly rinse the soaked buckwheat before combining with the soaked fruits and nuts.

An example of a great combination:
¼ cup buckwheat, 2 Tbsp. sunflower seeds, ¼ cup almonds, ¼ cup raisins, 3 dates, ½ banana (mashed), fresh berries.

Baked Oatmeal

1 1/2 cups steel cut oats
3/4 cup raisins
4 1/2 cups boiling water

1/4 tsp. sea salt
1/2 tsp. cinnamon
3 Tbsp. oil/butter

Combine all ingredients in casserole dish. Cover and bake at 350 degrees for 50-60 min. Serve topped with chopped nuts, blueberry sauce, banana milk, etc.

Cream of Rice Cereal

1 cup brown rice
3 cups water

¼ tsp. sea salt
opt: ½ cup raisins

Process rice in a blender until it is the consistency of coarse sand. Add water and sea salt (and raisins, if including) to a saucepan and bring to a boil. Whisk in the brown rice and simmer for 5- 8 minutes, stirring occasionally, until cereal is tender. Top with non-dairy milk and/or honey, agave or maple syrup.

Note: *Sometimes it works best to process 2 cups of rice at a time, to keep it circulating well in your blender. Store unused portion in refrigerator or freezer.*

Nut Milk

½ cup raw nuts (almonds, hazelnuts, etc.)
1+ Tbsp. sesame seeds   opt: 1-2 tsp. agave*
4 cups water   opt: pinch of sea salt

Soak nuts and seeds overnight. Drain then blend with rest of ingredients and strain through a fine sieve into a jar. Store in the refrigerator for 2-3 days.
*or honey or maple syrup

Banana Milk

1 1/2 banana (frozen)   2 Tbsp. flax oil
2 cups water   opt: 1 date
pinch sea salt

Puree in blender and use right away over muesli, buckwheat cereal, cooked cereal or fruit salad.

*This is our favorite milk alternative-
it's fast, easy and pleasantly sweet.*

Trail Mix/Snack Mix

almonds	raisins
walnuts	dates
sunflower seeds	other dried fruit
pumpkin seeds	(apples, apricots, etc.)

Mix equal portions of each *(or more of whatever you like best!)* and store in a container.

Great for taking on trips- from a simple
afternoon outing to a week-long vacation.
Keep some for 'emergencies' in a diaper bag,
carry-on bag or even in your glove compartment!

Nut-Stuffed Dates

Slice down length of date, without cutting in half, and remove pit. Insert two almonds, pecans or walnut halves into each date. These are also great stuffed with almond butter! For an added touch, the tops of stuffed dates can be pressed into coconut before being placed on a serving tray.

Simple, but such a tasty treat!
Great for the holidays, to serve to company or take to a party.

Fruit and Nut Balls

1 cup pitted dates
1 cup almonds
1 cup raisins
2 Tbsp. honey

1 tsp. pumpkin pie spice
   or cinnamon
1 Tbsp. orange zest
1/8 tsp. sea salt

Chop the nuts in the food processor, than add the rest of the ingredients and continue processing until finely chopped and the mixture begins holding together. Roll into balls and arrange on a platter. Additionally, each ball can be rolled in sesame seeds, shredded coconut, carob powder or chopped nuts. It makes an attractive presentation if the balls are rolled in an assortment of toppings.

*The combination of spices and orange zest in these fruit balls
conjures memories of the holidays.
They're really nice served at the holidays
and taken to parties.*

Gluten-free Baking Mixes

Why use a baking mix?

I actually don't like it when cookbooks similar to this one become dependent upon "mixes". Every recipe references back to a mix you were supposed to have prepared ahead and in most of these other books the mixes feature a fair bit of the refined gums, starches and flours I want to avoid. But I have worked on developing a few gluten-free blends as an option for those who enjoy having the convenience of a mix. It can be very handy for whipping up some muffins, biscuits, a cake or even a batch of pancakes. I offer a few different blends because even in the realm of gluten-free some people are avoiding one thing and another person is avoiding something else. For instance, when I wrote my first allergen-free baking booklet, I used an oat and buckwheat blend for most recipes. I still really like this blend and recommend it, yet even certified gluten-free oats can be problematic for some and also can be very costly, so I offer blends blends that don't include any oats. Another blend includes corn flour, which adds a nice unique texture and flavor, especially for toasted items, yet some people are allergic to corn. So I offer four blends for you to play around with, and a few simple recipes that use a gluten-free mix as a base. Please remember, I've developed these through trial and error and you can do the same, and perhaps arrive at something even better!

An immense variety of baked goods can be created by adding liquids, oil/butter and sweeteners to these basic mixes.

49

Ground almonds or sesame seeds can be substituted for some of the gluten-free flour in any of the mixes for an even richer baked good (experiment with amounts to find a flavor to your liking).

A number of the muffin recipes and cake recipes are made from flour blends similar to some of the baking mixes included here. I occasionally point this out in a note at the bottom of the recipe.

Simple recipes utilizing baking mixes are listed under each of the following four blends. The recipes are open-ended in that you can add any combination of spices and additions to them.

For sweetener, you can select from honey, agave or maple syrup.

For spices, you might select from cinnamon, nutmeg, ginger, cloves, cardamom, etc.

For additions, you could include any of the following:
> Applesauce (decrease amount of water for this option)
> Grated apples
> Chopped nuts
> Nut meal
> Blueberries or other berries
> Grated zucchini or carrot (decrease water with zucchini)
> Dried fruit
> Chocolate chips/carob chips

Basic Baking Mix *corn and oat free*

Single Recipe

1 cup brown rice flour

2/3 cup sorghum flour

1/3 cup light buckwheat flour

¼ cup ground flax

2 tsp. baking powder

¼-½ tsp. sea salt

Bulk Quantity (enough for about 4 recipes)

4 cups brown flour

2 2/3 cups sorghum flour

1 1/3 cups light buckwheat flour

1 cup ground flax

3 Tbsp. baking powder

1-2 tsp. sea salt

Mix and then store in the freezer to help prevent the natural oils in the grains and flax from oxidizing.

The advantage of this particular mix is that it contains no potential allergens (like corn and oats) or more difficult to find ingredients (like teff).

Baking Mix Pancakes

Add to 2 ¼ cups of your choice of baking mix:

2 1/4 cups water

1-2 Tbsp. honey

2 Tbsp. oil/butter

2 tsp. apple cider vinegar

Pour onto a medium skillet and cook until lightly browned on each side. (Flip when bubbles form on top of first side).

Oat Buckwheat Baking Mix

Single Recipe

1 3/4 cup GF oat flour

1/3 cup brown rice flour

1/3 cup light buckwheat flour

¼ cup ground flax

2 tsp. baking powder

¼-½ tsp. sea salt

Bulk Quantity (enough for about 4 recipes)

5 1/3 cups GF oat flour

1 1/3 cups brown rice flour

1 1/3 cups light buckwheat flour

1 cup ground flax

3 Tbsp. baking powder

1-2 tsp. sea salt

Mix and then store in the freezer to help prevent the natural oils in the grains and flax from oxidizing.

IMPORTANT NOTE: Because oat flour is so fine, include an additional ¼- 1/3 cup of this baking mix in recipes.

Baking Mix Biscuits

Add to 2 ¼ cups of your choice of baking mix:

1 1/2 cups of water

1-2 tsp. honey

Additional ½ tsp. sea salt

¼ cup oil/butter

1 tsp. apple cider vinegar

Additional 2 Tbsp. ground flax

Mix and allow to set for a minute or two before dropping on a baking sheet. Bake at 400 degrees for 15-18 minutes.

Corn Sorghum Baking Mix

Single Recipe

1 cup sorghum flour

1/2 cup corn flour

1/2 cup brown rice flour

¼ cup ground flax

2 tsp. baking powder

¼-½ tsp. sea salt

Bulk Quantity (enough for about 4 recipes)

4 cups sorghum flour

2 cups corn flour

2 cups brown rice flour

1 cup ground flax

3 Tbsp. baking powder

1-2 tsp. sea salt

Mix and then store in the freezer to help prevent the natural oils in the grains and flax from oxidizing.

Baking Mix Muffins

Add to 2 ¼ cups of your choice of baking mix:

1 cup water

½ cup applesauce

1/3 cup sweetener*

Up to 1 ½ tsp. spice*

¼ cup oil/butter

1 tsp. apple cider vinegar

Additional 2 Tbsp. ground flax

Up to 1 cup additions*

Bake in muffin cups at 400 degrees for 18-20 minutes.

*See page 50 for possible options.

Oat Rice Baking Mix

Single Recipe

2/3 cup GF oat flour

2/3 cup brown rice flour

1/3 cup sorghum flour

1/3 cup light buckwheat flour

¼ cup ground flax

2 tsp. baking powder

¼-½ tsp. sea salt

Bulk Quantity (enough for about 4 recipes)

2 2/3 cup GF oat flour

2 2/3 cup brown rice flour

1 1/3 cup sorghum flour

1 1/3 cup light buckwheat flour

1 cup ground flax

3 Tbsp. baking powder

¼-½ tsp. sea salt

Mix and then store in the freezer to help prevent the natural oils in the grains and flax from oxidizing.

Baking Mix Cake

Add to 2 ½ cups of your choice of baking mix:

1 1/3 cup water

4 Tbsp. oil/butter

Opt: up to 1 ½ tsp. spice

½- 2/3 cup sweetener*

1 tsp. apple cider vinegar

Opt: 1-2 cups of additions*

Bake in an 8 ½ x 11 pan at 350 degrees for 45-50 minutes.
*See page 50 for possible options.
Variation: add streusel topping (pg. 34) for coffee cake!

Quick Biscuits

1 cup sorghum flour
1/3 cup light buckwheat flour
1/3 cup cornmeal
1/3 cup brown rice flour
2 tsp. baking powder
1/2+ tsp. sea salt

1 1/3 cup warm water
3 Tbsp. oil/butter
1/3 cup ground flax
1 tsp. apple cider vinegar
1 tsp. honey*

Combine wet ingredients (right column) in a mixing bowl or shake together in a sealed canning jar. Mix dry ingredients (in left column) together in another bowl (adding any of the optional additions from below). Lightly combine with wet ingredients, being careful to not overmix. Pat dough out onto a floured surface until it is about ½ inch thick. Cut into rounds (the top of a drinking glass works well for this purpose) or drop biscuits by spoon or ice cream scoop onto baking sheet. Bake at 400 degrees for about 15-18 minutes, until lightly browned. Line sheet with parchment paper for easy clean-up.

* or agave or maple syrup

Optional additional dry ingredients-
1/2 tsp. dried herbs (dill, oregano, parsley)
1 tsp. onion or garlic powder
2 tsp. dried chives
1-4 Tbsp. seeds (sesame, poppy, sunflower)

Oat Biscuits

2 cups GF oat flour*
2 tsp. baking powder
1/2+ tsp. sea salt

1/3 cup ground flax
3 Tbsp. oil/butter
3/4- 1 cup warm water

Combine wet ingredients (right column). I like to shake them together in a sealed canning jar. Mix dry ingredients together in a bowl (adding any of the optional additions from below). Add wet ingredients to dry and lightly mix together. Drop onto baking sheet and bake at 400 degrees for about 20 minutes, until lightly browned.

* easily ground from gluten-free rolled or steel cut oats if you don't have gluten-free oat flour on hand.

Optional: any of the optional ingredients from the quick biscuits recipe can be added to these biscuits as well.

Shortcake Biscuits

To Oat Biscuit recipe (above), add:

     1/3 cup ground almond meal
     1 Tbsp. of water
     up to 2 Tbsp. honey (opt.)

Then prepare and bake according to the above directions.

These are great topped with chopped fresh fruit or fruit sauce.

Oat Scones

1 cup GF rolled oats

1 ½ cup GF oat flour

½ cup almond meal*

1 Tbsp. baking powder

½ tsp. sea salt

½ cup non-dairy milk

1/3 cup oil/butter

3 Tbsp. ground flax

2 Tbsp. honey

opt.: ½ cup currants/raisins

In a large bowl, mix together dry ingredients (in left column). Combine wet ingredients (right column). Add wet to dry and mix just till moistened (avoid over-mixing). Take half of the dough and pat it into a circle on a baking sheet or stone (oiled or lined with parchment paper) about 1" thick and 8 inches across. Do likewise with other half of dough. Cut each circle into 8 wedges (4 cuts)- a pizza cutter works great for this. Bake at 425 degrees for about 15 minutes, till tops are lightly browned.

* Almond meal can be made from whole almonds by processing in a sturdy blender or coffee grinder.

Cornbread

1 cup cornmeal
1/2 cup brown rice flour
1/2 cup sorghum flour
2 tsp. baking powder
3/4 tsp. sea salt

1 1/4 cup water
1 tsp. apple cider vinegar
3 Tbsp. oil/butter
2+ Tbsp. honey
1/4 cup ground flax

Combine dry ingredients (in left column) in a mixing bowl. Whisk together the wet ingredients (right column) and then mix lightly with the dry ingredients. Pour into an oiled 8 ½ x 11 rectangular baking pan and bake at 400 degrees for about 22-25 minutes.

Also great baked in cast iron skillet.

Excellent served with soup or chili.

Basic Bread

1 cup brown rice flour
2/3 cup sorghum flour
1/3 cup cornmeal
1 Tbsp. baking powder

1 3/4 cup water
1/2 cup ground flax
2 Tbsp. oil/butter
3/4 -1 tsp. sea salt
1 tsp. honey or agave
1 tsp. apple cider vinegar

Mix dry ingredients (left column) in a mixing bowl. Combine wet ingredients (right column- *I like to shake them together in a sealed canning jar*). Lightly mix together with a spoon or spatula and then pour into an oiled loaf pan. Bake at 350 degrees for 45-50 minutes. Allow for the bread to "rest" for at least ½ hour before attempting to slice.

This resembles more traditional slicing bread,
with a tender biscuit-like flavor.
It's really great toasted!

Blender Bread

1 cup brown rice
3/4 cup millet*
Opt: 2 Tbsp. sesame seeds
1 Tbsp. apple cider vinegar
_____
½ cup cornmeal
2 tsp. baking powder
½ tsp. baking soda

1 ¼ cup water
2 Tbsp. oil/butter
1 Tbsp. honey**
2 tsp. apple cider vinegar
¼ cup ground flax
1 tsp. sea salt

Soak ingredients above line in left column in plenty of water for at least 8 hours (or overnight). Drain well then add with ingredients in right column in a blender and blend until smooth. Combine last three ingredients (below line in left column). Sift through a sieve and whisk into bread batter to avoid lumps. Pour into an oiled loaf pan and bake at 350 degrees for about 55 minutes. Allow to cool for at least ½ an hour before attempting to slice.

*or a combination of millet and buckwheat groats
**or agave or maple syrup

This bread holds together well and is great sliced and toasted!
Excellent for sandwich-making.

Grilled cheese sandwich: Grill sliced bread with butter and then spread with Cheese Sauce (pg.70). *Gluten and casein-free!*

Banana Bread

1 cup brown rice flour	3-4 bananas, mashed
3/4 cup teff flour*	1/4 cup oil/butter
2 tsp. baking powder	1/4 cup water
1/2 tsp. baking soda	1/4 cup honey/molasses
1/4 tsp. sea salt	1 tsp. apple cider vinegar
1 tsp. cinnamon	1/2 cup ground flax
opt: 1/4 tsp. cardamom	3/4 cup chopped nuts**
	opt: 1/2 raisins

Mix ingredients in left column in a mixing bowl. Combine wet ingredients (in right column) and then mix lightly with the dry ingredients. Pour into an oiled loaf pan and bake at 350 degrees for about 50 minutes.

* or sorghum or light buckwheat flour
** walnuts or pecans

This bread is delicious! It was one of the first gluten-free recipes I developed and I found the flavor and texture so good, I began to wonder "What's the big deal with gluten-free?!" When it tastes this good and is this good for us, it certainly makes it a lot easier to leave traditional gluten-containing foods behind!

Zucchini Bread

1 cup brown rice flour
2/3 cup sorghum flour
1/3 cup light buckwheat flour
1 tsp. baking powder
1 tsp. baking soda
½-1 tsp. sea salt
2 tsp. cinnamon
½ tsp. nutmeg

2 cups grated zucchini
1/2 cup applesauce
1/3 cup oil/butter
1/3 cup ground flax
2/3 cup honey*
¼ cup water
1 tsp. apple cider vinegar
¾ cup chopped nuts
opt.: ½ cup raisins

Mix dry ingredients in left column. Mix wet ingredients in right column (all but nuts and raisins), then combine with dry ingredients. Fold in nuts and raisins, if including. Pour into an oiled loaf pan and bake at 350 degrees for at least 1 hour. (Test with a toothpick or knife). Allow to cool for at least 20 minutes before slicing.

* or agave or maple syrup

Great toasted!

Brown Bread

¾ cup corn meal

1 ¼ cup boiling water

2 Tbsp. oil/butter

2 Tbsp. apple cider vinegar

½ cup ground flax

1/3- 1/2 cup molasses*

3 Tbsp. honey**

1 ¼ cup sorghum flour

1 tsp. baking soda

2 tsp. baking powder

1 tsp. sea salt

¾ cup raisins

Whisk cornmeal into boiling water in a large mixing bowl. Allow to set for 10-15 minutes before adding the rest of the ingredients in the left column. Mix ingredients in the right column in separate bowl and then combine briefly, but thoroughly, into the wet mixture (you'll see a neat reaction!). Pour into an oiled loaf pan and bake at 350 degrees for 50-55 minutes. Allow to cool for at least ½ hour before attempting to slice.

* there are different "intensities" of molasses, so adjust the amount according to your taste

** or agave or maple syrup

*Traditionally called "Boston Brown Bread"
and served with baked beans,
my grandmother made some of the best around!*

Flatbread

1/2 cup light buckwheat flour	1 cup warm water
1/2 cup corn flour	2 Tbsp. olive oil
1/2 cup sorghum flour	1 Tbsp. apple cider vinegar
1/2 cup GF oat flour	opt: 1 tsp. agave or honey
1/2 cup teff flour	1 tsp. sea salt
1/3 cup ground flax	1 tsp. baking powder
	up to 1/2 cup flour of choice

Combine ingredients in left column. Mix together water, oil, vinegar, (honey or agave) and sea salt, then combine well with flour mixture. Allow to rest for about 1 hour. Preheat baking stones in a 550 degree oven. Mix baking powder into your choice of flour and then mix a small amount into the original mixture until it begins to hold together well (such that you can roll it out onto the counter and begin kneading it). Knead for a few minutes, adding flour as necessary, to prevent it from sticking. Cut into about sixteen pieces. Roll or pat each piece into a flatbread, about 1/8" thick. I like using a little cornmeal on the countertop at this stage. Toss each piece onto a preheated baking sheet or stone. Bake for about 7-8 minutes. It will lightly brown and may puff up slightly.

Optional: add some garlic powder to dough and/or pat some sesame seeds into the flatbreads before baking.

Variation: this recipe calls for a blend of several flours, but you can substitute any of the flours with good results.

Crackers

2 cups sorghum flour*	1 1/4 cup warm water
2/3 cup teff flour**	1/3 cup ground flax
1/2 cup cornmeal	1 Tbsp. oil/butter
3 Tbsp. sesame seeds	1 Tbsp. molasses
2 tsp. baking powder	2 tsp. apple cider vinegar
1 1/4 tsp. sea salt	opt: 1/2 tsp. garlic powder

Mix dry ingredients (left column). Combine wet ingredients (right column) and then mix with flour mixture into a dry dough. Cut into two pieces. Lightly roll each half in flour. Pat onto a baking stone (or baking sheet lined with parchment paper). Sprinkle each half with ½ of the seed mixture (below) and gently roll into dough, until dough is about ¼ inch thick. (The seeds work well to prevent the dough from sticking to the rolling pin). Prick surface with a fork, then cut into squares or rectangles with a pizza cutter. Bake at 350 degrees for about 30 minutes (until lightly browned) then another ½ hour or more at 200 degrees to get them nice and crisp. Ideally leave in the oven overnight. Cool before packing.

* or light buckwheat flour
** or part brown rice flour and light buckwheat flour

Seed topping:

½ cup sunflower seeds	¼ cup flax seeds
¼ cup sesame seeds	opt: 2 Tbsp. poppy seeds

Ranch Dressing

1 ¼ cup sunflower seeds
juice of 2 lemons (about 1/3- ½ cup)
1 clove garlic
2 Tbsp. tahini
1 ½ tsp. sea salt
½ tsp. onion powder

1 ¾ cup water
1/3 cup oil
¾ tsp. basil
½ tsp. oregano
½ tsp. thyme

PREP: Presoak sunflower seeds for at least 6 hours.

Blend ingredients in left column with water in right column. When smooth, gently blend in oil and herbs. This dressing is best if made ahead, so the herbs are allowed time to contribute their flavor.

This dressing is excellent on salad, but we especially enjoy it on salad pockets made with lentil cakes. You gotta' try this!

Creamy Dill Dressing

Make "Ranch Dressing" above and substitute 1 Tbsp. dried dill weed for the other herbs.

Almond Mayonnaise

1 cup almonds

¾ cup water

juice of 1 lemon (about 1/4 cup)

1 tsp. apple cider vinegar

Opt: 1 tsp. honey or agave

¾ tsp. onion powder

¼ tsp. mustard powder

1 ½ - 2 tsp. sea salt

1 cup olive/flax oil

PREP: Presoak almonds for at least 8 hours.

Drain and rinse almonds. Puree all ingredients in blender, except for oil. When mixture is quite smooth, gently blend in oil (adding more water, if necessary, to reach correct consistency).

Optional: For a light-colored mayonnaise, peel almonds before adding to blender.

Store in refrigerator for up to one week.

Sunflower Sour Cream

3/4 cup sunflower seeds
juice of 1 lemon (about 1/4 cup)
½ cup water*
1 Tbsp. olive oil

1/2 tsp. sea salt
1 tsp. onion powder
1/4 tsp. garlic powder

Ideally, presoak sunflower seeds for at least 6 hours.** Drain and then blend with the rest of the ingredients until smooth. Refrigerate and use within a few days.

* add more water for a thinner consistency.

** if you haven't presoaked the sunflower seeds, add an additional ½ cup water to mixture.

Great served on baked potatoes or with Mexican dishes.

Pesto Sauce

4 large garlic cloves

1 cup fresh basil leaves

1 Tbsp. lemon juice

1/2 tsp. sea salt

1/3 cup olive oil

opt: 1/3 cup pinenuts.

Blend garlic, basil, lemon juice and unrefined sea salt in food processor until it forms a paste. Slowly mix in olive oil. Serve over pasta, rice or steamed vegetables and sprinkle with pine nuts.

Extra sauce can be frozen in ice cube trays,
then stored in the freezer for up to 3 months

Pasta and Grain Salads

Pasta salads can successfully be made with gluten-free pasta. Prepare as you would with traditional pasta.

Cooked quinoa and brown rice work great in cold salads. Simply chill and then mix with raw or steamed veggies plus salad dressing, oil and lemon, or pesto sauce (recipe above).

Cheese Sauce

1 2/3 cup water	1 Tbsp. lemon juice
1/3 cup GF rolled oats*	1 tsp. onion powder
1/3 cup nutritional yeast	½ tsp. ground mustard
2 Tbsp. tahini	¼ tsp. garlic powder
1 ½ tsp. sea salt	¼ tsp. turmeric
3 Tbsp. oil/butter	¼ tsp. paprika
opt: ½ tsp. basil	opt: ½ tsp. parsley

Combine ingredients in a blender and blend until smooth. Bring to a boil in a saucepan, then simmer on low until thickened- whisking frequently.

*Or ¼ cup sorghum flour or brown rice flour. If you are using flour in place of the oats, the ingredients can be whisked together in a saucepan (no need to blend them before adding to the saucepan)

To make a "sharper" cheese, add more tahini and lemon juice.

This amount of sauce is perfect for topping one pound of pasta. It also makes a great topping for nachos and baked potatoes.

Hummus

15 oz. can chickpeas (drained)* 1-2 cloves of garlic
1/2 tsp. unrefined sea salt juice of 1 lemon (1/4 cup)
1/8 tsp. ground cumin 2-3 Tbsp. tahini
1 tsp. olive oil

Puree everything in food processor until smooth, adding some liquid from canned beans if too thick. Before serving, drizzle with olive oil and sprinkle with paprika.
* or 2 cups cooked chickpeas/garbanzo beans

Optional: The amount of lemon juice, garlic, tahini and salt can be adjusted to your taste.

Serve with cut veggies and/or tortilla chips.
Crackers (page 65) also go great with this dip.

Makes an excellent contribution to parties and potlucks.

Herbed White Gravy

3 Tbsp. oil/butter
5 Tbsp. brown rice flour*
1 Tbsp. onion powder
¼ tsp. garlic powder
Opt: 1 Tbsp. dried parsley

½ tsp. poultry seasoning
½ tsp. thyme
1 tsp. salt
2 ½ cups water and/or
    non-dairy milk**

In a saucepan, sauté flour in oil until bubbly. Add rest of ingredients, whisking together. Heat until thickened.
*or 5 Tbsp. sorghum flour or ½ cup GF rolled oats. If using GF oats, blend all ingredients in blender (except for oil/butter and herbs) and then simmer with oil/butter and herbsin saucepan until thickened, or grind the oats into flour before preparing as described above.
** we usually prepare this gravy with half water/half "milk". Be sure the non-dairy milk you use for this purpose isn't sweetened.

Onion Gravy

Prepare Herbed White Gravy as above except sauté 2 thinly sliced onions in oil/butter before adding flour to the saucepan.

*Both gravies are great on biscuits,
baked potatoes and veggies.*

Green Salads

*Having a **variety** of salad components on hand*
keeps salads changing and interesting

The salad base- a combination of:

> green leaf, red leaf or romaine lettuce
>
> spinach leaves, mesclun, baby greens
>
> small pieces of kale, endive, other "exotic" greens
>
> thinly sliced green or red cabbage

The usual toppings:

carrot, grated or sliced	red/sweet onion
cucumbers	tomatoes
red/yellow bell peppers	celery
	radishes

A little more out of the ordinary:

zucchini	sprouts
cauliflower	yellow squash
green peas	broccoli
beets, grated raw	avocado
marinated tomatoes	marinated veggies
herbs- parsley, basil, cilantro, chives, etc.	

Getting a little "out there":

snow peas	jicama
broccoli stalks, diced	kohlrabi
raw corn from cob	fennel
scallions	Jerusalem artichokes
daikon radish	chickpeas
kidney, other beans	salsa, hummus
chili, crumbled tortilla chips	guacamole

73

Crunchy, flavorful and nutritional additions:

nuts- walnuts, almonds, pecans, pine nuts, etc.

seeds- sunflower, pumpkin, sesame, etc.

ground flax seed   vegetarian bacon bits

flax oil   dried fruit (raisins, etc.)

. . . and dressing, of course!

Salad-Making Tips

Salad spinners and a **food processor** (or salad shooter) are really helpful in salad-making.

We try to keep a **"salad bar"** handy in our refrigerator-

We make up a **salad base** (enough for a few days),

or at least have prewashed lettuce ready.

Then we just chop, grate, or cut up a **new veggie** or two each day (more than for just one meal).

We also keep a **tray of toppings** (seeds, nuts, oils, sprinkles, dressing) handy in the refrigerator.

Some people prefer making up a fresh salad each evening with their food processor (fast prep!).

Serve coleslaw, spinach salad, grated vegetable salads, cut veggies and dip, or other raw veggie dishes in place of green salad on occasion, so everyone can enjoy the variety.

Black Bean and Quinoa Salad

3 cups boiling water

1 1/2 cups quinoa

2 cans black beans

1 lb. pkg. baby peas

½ cup finely chopped sweet onion*

1/3 cup olive oil

2 ½ Tbsp. vinegar**

6 Tbsp. lemon juice

1 ½ tsp. sea salt

½ cup chopped parsley

1 cup chopped cilantro

Rinse quinoa thoroughly, then combine with boiling water and cook, covered, for 18-20 minutes. Lightly steam baby peas. Allow both to cool.

Combine oil, vinegar, lemon juice and sea salt in a large bowl. Mix in quinoa, black beans, peas and herbs. Toss gently to blend. Serve at room temperature.

* or 4 scallions

** raw apple cider vinegar

This salad is a wonderful alternative to traditional pasta salads. It makes a large portion and can be enjoyed over several days. My oldest son says that he could live on this salad!

Pizza Crust

1 ¼ cup brown rice flour
¾ cup cornmeal/corn flour*
1 ½ cup warm/hot water
3 Tbsp. ground flax
2 Tbsp. olive oil
1 Tbsp. apple cider vinegar

1 ½ tsp. sea salt
1 tsp. agave or honey

_____

½+ cup sorghum flour**
2 tsp. baking powder

Preheat oven to 425 degrees and preheat baking stones or cast iron skillets.

Combine all ingredients, except for the sorghum flour and baking powder, in a mixing bowl. Allow to set for at least one hour before mixing in the last two ingredients. (If you're short on time, use boiling water and allow to the mixture to sit for just a few minutes before adding flour and baking powder.)

Dust surface of baking stone with sesame seeds or cornmeal or oil cast iron skillet with 1 Tbsp.+ of olive oil. Divide dough into two portions and press onto stone or into skillet or use full amount for a thick crust or deep dish pizza.

Bake crust for about 10 minutes, top with sauce and toppings, then bake for another 10-15 minutes.

* sorghum flour can also be used, though we prefer the corn
** or light buckwheat flour

Makes enough batter for two thin crust pizzas or one thick crust. This recipe produces a "biscuit-style" crust.

Blender Pizza Crust

1 cup brown rice

½ cup millet

1 Tbsp. apple cider vinegar

_____

½ cup corn meal/corn flour

2 tsp. baking powder

½ tsp. baking soda

1 ¼ cup water

1 tsp. agave or honey

1 tsp. apple cider vinegar

2 Tbsp. ground flax

2 Tbsp. olive oil

1 ½ tsp. sea salt

Soak the brown rice and millet with vinegar in water for at least 6-8 hours (ideally, overnight).

Preheat oven to 425 degrees and preheat baking stones or cast iron skillets. The baking stones work great for thin pizza and the skillet for thin or deep-dish style.

Drain the soaked grains well and then process with the ingredients in the right column. Separately combine the cornmeal/flour, baking powder and soda. Sift through a sieve and whisk into processed batter to avoid lumps.

Dust surface of baking stone with sesame seeds or cornmeal, or oil cast iron skillet with 1 Tbsp.+ of olive oil. Pour batter in thin layer onto hot baking stone (shake a little to level) or into a deep dish-style layer in the preheated cast iron skillet.

Bake crust for about 10 minutes, top with sauce and toppings, then bake for another 10-15 minutes.

Makes enough batter for two pizzas.

Besides being more nutritious and beneficial being made from soaked grains, this pizza crust recipe is wonderful because you don't have to roll or press the dough out. Just pour on and cook!

The thin crust has a nice cracker-like texture.
The thick crust has a nice light deep-dish quality.

This pizza reheats well in an oven or toaster oven.

Quick Pizza Sauce

1 Tbsp. olive oil
2 cloves garlic, crushed
pinch cayenne
1/4 tsp. sea salt

8 oz. tomato sauce
2 tsp. oregano
1/2 tsp. basil
1/2 tsp. thyme

Sauté garlic in oil. Add rest of ingredients. Simmer for at least 15 minutes, until the sauce begins to thicken.

Variation: Sauté one chopped onion with the garlic.

Pasta and Sauce

Pasta is traditionally made from wheat, yet many excellent gluten-free pastas are now commonly available. You can also use cooked spaghetti squash or spiral-sliced raw zucchini as a base for pasta and sauce- with greater nutritional value too! Also try topped with pesto (pg. 69).

Tomato (Marinara) Sauce

2 Tbsp. olive/coconut oil

1 onion, chopped

3-4 cloves garlic, crushed

1/4 tsp. chili powder

1/2 tsp. unrefined sea salt

opt: 1/2 red pepper, chopped

      5-6 mushrooms, sliced

28 oz. canned tomatoes

1 tsp. basil

1 tsp. oregano

1 Tbsp. parsley

opt: pinch cayenne

Sauté onion and garlic (peppers, mushrooms) in oil. Add rest of ingredients and simmer for at least 30 minutes, up to 2 hours.

Serve over gluten-free pasta, brown rice, beans, and/or steamed or sautéed vegetables.

Chili

2 Tbsp. oil/butter	pinch cayenne
3-4 onions, chopped	1 1/2 tsp. sea salt
6 cloves garlic, crushed	28 oz. can tomatoes
2 Tbsp. chili powder	5 cans/7 cups beans
2 tsp. oregano	(lightly drained)
2 tsp. cumin	-kidney, cannellini,
1/2 tsp. cinnamon	black beans, etc.

Sauté onions and garlic in oil, add seasonings, then tomatoes and beans. Bring to a boil then simmer for at least 20 minutes, stirring occasionally.

Optional: Add 1 diced bell pepper and/or 2 cups corn.

*Great served with brown rice, cornbread
or just tortilla chips and salsa.*

*Leftover chili is great reheated with some cornbread
or used to top salads or baked potatoes.*

*Chili makes a great company meal and potluck contribution.
It's one of my most popular dishes!*

Versatile Mexican Meal

Any combination of the following components can be wrapped in a gluten-free wrap, folded into a corn tortilla or layered into a "bean and rice bowl" or "taco salad". This meal will easily become a family favorite!

Refried beans

Black beans

Pintos

Brown rice

Sautéed onions/peppers

Grilled zucchini/squash

Corn

Salsa

Guacamole

Shredded lettuce

Diced tomatoes

Diced bell pepper

Diced onion

Sliced avocado

Sliced black olives

Chopped cilantro

Sunflower Sour Cream (page 68)

Cheese Sauce (page 70)

Gingerbread Cake

1 cup teff flour*

1/3 cup light buckwheat flour

1 Tbsp. cinnamon

2 tsp. ground ginger

½ tsp. ground cloves

1 tsp. baking powder

1 tsp. baking soda

½ tsp. sea salt

¾ cup warm water

1/3 cup oil/butter

½ cup molasses**

¼ cup honey***

1 cup applesauce

2 tsp. apple cider vinegar

½ cup ground flax

¾ cup brown rice flour

Combine wet ingredients (right column, including brown rice flour), allowing the mixture to set for several minutes for the brown rice flour to hydrate. Combine dry ingredients (left column) in a mixing bowl. Combine wet and dry mixtures and then pour into an oiled 8 ½ x 11 rectangular baking pan. Bake at 350 degrees for 35-40 minutes.

* or sorghum flour

** increase depending upon intensity of molasses

***or agave or maple syrup

Fancy Version:

Make this an "Upside Down Cake" by layering the bottom of the cake pan with thinly sliced pears or apples before pouring in the cake batter. It's really special when baked in a cast-iron skillet. Scrumptious, and a beautiful autumn presentation!

Coffee Cake

2 ½ cups baking mix*
1 ½ tsp. cinnamon
¼ tsp. nutmeg
1 cup chopped walnuts
Streusel Topping (pg. 34)

1 1/3 cup water
¼ cup oil/butter
½- 2/3 cup honey**
1 tsp. apple cider vinegar

Mix ingredients in left column in a large bowl. Combine wet ingredients (right column) and then mix with dry ingredients. Pour into an oiled 8 ½ x 11 baking pan. Crumble or drizzle "Streusel Topping" over top and then bake at 350 degrees for 45-50 minutes.

* any blend except for "Corn Sorghum Baking Mix" will work well for this cake.

** agave or maple syrup

This cake is an example of how
the Baking Mix Cake recipe (page 54) can be used.

Spiced Apple Cake

1 cup brown rice flour
2/3 cup GF oat flour
1/3 cup light buckwheat flour
1 cup GF rolled oats
1 Tbsp. cinnamon
½ tsp. nutmeg
Opt: ¼ tsp. cloves
1 tsp. baking powder
1 tsp. baking soda
½ tsp. sea salt

2/3 cup water
½ cup honey*
¼ cup oil/butter
1 cup applesauce
2 tsp. lemon juice
1/3 cup ground flax
3 cups chopped apples

opt: 1 cup chopped nuts
opt: 1 cup raisins

Mix dry ingredients (left column) in a bowl. Mix wet ingredients (right column) and then lightly combine with dry ingredients. Pour into an oiled 8 ½ x 11 rectangular baking pan. Bake at 350 degrees for 50-55 minutes.

* or agave or maple syrup

Carrot Cake

1 cup brown rice flour	½ -2/3 cup honey*
2/3 cup sorghum flour	1/3 cup oil/butter
1/3 light buckwheat flour	1 cup crushed pineapple
2 tsp. baking powder	2 cups finely grated carrots
1 tsp. baking soda	½-1 cup applesauce
½ tsp. sea salt	2/3 cup water
1 Tbsp. cinnamon	1 tsp. apple cider vinegar
½ tsp. ground ginger	½ cup ground flax
¼ tsp. allspice	1 cup chopped nuts
opt: ¾ cup raisins	opt: ¾ cup shredded coconut

Mix dry ingredients in left column. Mix wet ingredients in right column and combine with dry ingredients. Pour into an oiled 8 ½ x 11 rectangular baking pan and bake at 350 degrees for about 50 minutes.

* or agave or maple syrup

This cake has a lot of special additions- pineapple, raisins, nuts, and coconut. Feel free to leave out any you'd like, just be sure to add a little more water or applesauce if you leave out the crushed pineapple. More applesauce makes it moister.

The flour blend in this recipe is the same
as the Basic Baking Mix.
The cake is also great made with the
Oat Buckwheat Baking Mix blend.

Chocolate Cake

1 cup brown rice flour

1 cup sorghum flour*

1 ½ tsp. baking powder

1 tsp. baking soda

½- ¾ tsp. sea salt

2 1/2 cups boiling water

1 cup cocoa powder

½ cup applesauce

½ cup oil/butter

2/3- ¾ cup honey**

1 Tbsp. apple cider vinegar

½ cup ground flax

Combine ingredients in left column in a large bowl. Whisk together the ingredients in the right column, then combine with the dry mixture. Pour into an oiled 8 ½ x 11 rectangular baking pan and bake at 350 degrees for about 45 minutes (until knife inserted in the center comes out clean).

* or 2/3 cup sorghum flour and 1/3 cup light buckwheat flour

** or agave or maple syrup, or a combination of these

Variation: soak ½ cup of pitted prunes in the 2 ½ cups boiling water, then process in a blender with the rest of the ingredients in the right column. This addition increases the depth of flavor plus moistness and nutritional value of the cake.

*This is cake is so tasty and moist
that it is great plain or topped with icing/frosting.
Decrease water by ¼ to 1/3 cup if you prefer a drier cake.*

Coconut Caramel Topping

½ cup oil/butter

½ cup honey

2 Tbsp. non-dairy milk

pinch of sea salt

1+ cup shredded coconut

1 cup chopped walnuts

Simmer all ingredients (except for coconut and walnuts) for several minutes- until the mixture begins to caramelize- stirring frequently. Stir in walnuts and coconut.

Spread on top of a baked cake. Place under broiler for a couple minutes (watch carefully), until it lightly browns.

This is particularly great on carrot cake and chocolate cake!

Cocoa-Coconut Frosting

1 1/2 cup non-dairy milk

1/4 cup brown rice flour

3 Tbsp. oil/butter

1/4 cup honey*

1 Tbsp. cocoa powder

1/3 cup shredded coconut

Combine all ingredients in saucepan and simmer until thickened. Allow to cool before frosting cake.

* or agave or maple syrup

Super on chocolate cake!

Oatmeal Chocolate Chip Cake

1 cup GF rolled oats
6 Tbsp. oil/butter
2 ¼ cups hot water
½-2/3 cup honey
¼ cup ground flax
1 cup brown rice flour

3/4 cup GF oat flour
1 Tbsp. cocoa powder
1 tsp. baking soda
1/2 tsp. sea salt
1 ¼- 1 ½ cup chocolate chips*
3/4 cup chopped walnuts

Pour hot water over rolled oats and oil/butter in a large bowl. Let set for about 10 minutes before whisking in the honey and ground flax. Mix the dry ingredients together, and then combine with the wet. Gently fold in about half of the chocolate chips. Pour into a rectangular cake pan. Sprinkle the rest of the chocolate chips plus the chopped walnuts on top. Bake at 350 degrees for 35-40 minutes.
*about 12 ounces

Carob version: substitute carob powder for cocoa powder and carob chips for chocolate chips.

Our family prefers the smaller amount of honey, since the chocolate chips themselves lend a fair bit of sweetness to the cake.

Blender Pineapple Cake

1 1/3 cup brown rice
2/3 cup millet (or ½ millet and
    raw buckwheat groats
1 Tbsp. apple cider vinegar
_____
20 oz. can crushed pineapple
2 Tbsp. oil/butter
¼ cup maple syrup

¼ cup oil/butter
1/3+ cup honey*
1 tsp. lemon juice
½ tsp. sea salt
1/3 cup ground flax
1/3 cup sorghum flour**
1 ½ tsp. baking powder
½ tsp. baking soda

Soak rice and millet (and buckwheat) in water and vinegar overnight (or for at least 8 hours). Preheat oven to 350 degrees. Drain pineapple in a colander, reserving pineapple juice. Combine the crushed pineapple, the 2 Tbsp. oil/butter and 1/4 cup maple syrup in the bottom of an 8 ½ x 11 rectangular baking pan. Place in oven to heat while preparing the cake batter.

Combine the pineapple juice with enough water to make 1 ¼ cups liquid total. Add the honey, lemon, salt, ground flax and the drained grains to a blender. Process until smooth. Whisk in the sorghum flour, baking powder and baking soda, then pour over top of pineapple mixture in cake pan. Bake at 350 degrees for about 45 minutes. Allow to cool for a few minutes before serving, or gently flip onto a serving platter for a nice presentation as an "upside down cake".

* or agave or maple syrup, use more if desired
** or light buckwheat flour

Banana Oat Cookies

2-3 ripe bananas, mashed
1/4 cup oil/butter
2 Tbsp. ground flax
1/4 tsp. sea salt
opt: ½ cup chopped nuts

1 ½ cup GF rolled oats
½ cup GF oat flour
1 tsp. cinnamon
½ cup raisins
opt: ¼ cup coconut

Combine wet ingredients in left column (mash them together on a plate or blend together in a blender). Mix dry ingredients (right column) and then combine with wet. Drop by spoonful onto a baking sheet. Bake at 375 degrees for 15-18 minutes (until lightly browned).

These cookies are neat in that they include no added sweetener and use very little oil.

Coconut Blender Cookies

1 cup brown rice
1/3 cup millet
1 Tbsp. apple cider vinegar
_____

4 cups shredded coconut
1 ½ tsp. baking powder

1 cup water
¾ cup honey*
3 Tbsp. oil/butter
1/3 cup ground flax
½ tsp. sea salt

Soak brown rice and millet with vinegar at least 8 hours (or overnight). Drain and rinse, then combine with ingredients in right column and blend until smooth. Combine coconut and baking powder in a large bowl, then mix in blender batter. Mound by teaspoon onto a baking sheet and bake at 350 degrees for about 22-25 minutes, till lightly browned (like a nice macaroon!). ***Makes 4-5 dozen cookies***

* or agave or maple syrup

Spiced Coconut Cookies: add 1 tsp. cinnamon, ¼ tsp. each of nutmeg, ginger and allspice to blender mixture. Just ¾ tsp. nutmeg on its own is really great too.

Chocolate Coconut Cookies: add ½ cup cocoa to blender mixture.

Chocolate Mint Cookies

1 cup teff flour*
½ cup sorghum flour**
¼ cup light buckwheat flour
2/3 cup cocoa powder
1 ½ tsp. baking powder
½ tsp. baking soda
½ tsp. sea salt

½ cup oil/butter
½- 2/3 cup honey***
1 cup water
1 tsp. apple cider vinegar
1/2 cup ground flax
½ tsp. peppermint extract
opt: 1 cup chopped nuts
opt: ½ chocolate chips

Combine dry ingredients (left column) in a mixing bowl. Combine wet ingredients (right column, except for optional ingredients) and then mix well with dry mixture. Either drop by teaspoon onto baking sheet or roll into a log in parchment paper and refrigerate for at least one hour before cutting into ½" slices and placing on baking sheet. Bake at 350 degrees for 15-18 minutes.

* or brown rice flour
**or GF oat flour
***or agave or maple syrup

Optional: flatten cookies with a spatula halfway through baking time

Carob version: replace cocoa powder with carob powder, chocolate chips with carob chips and add 2 Tbsp. tahini and 1 Tbsp. molasses to the batter.

Chocolate Chip Cookies

½ cup oil/butter
½ cup honey*
1/3 cup water
¼ cup ground flax
Opt: 1-2 tsp. vanilla

2 ¼ cup GF flour blend
1 tsp. baking soda
¾ tsp. sea salt
¾- 1 cup chocolate chips
opt: 1 cup chopped nuts

Mix wet ingredients (left column). Mix dry ingredients (right column, except for chocolate chips and nuts). Combine wet and dry and then mix in the chips (and nuts, if using). Drop by teaspoon onto a baking sheet (use parchment paper for easy clean-up) and bake at 350 degrees for 12-15 minutes. Allow to rest 5-10 minutes on baking sheets before transferring to cooking racks (will hold together better).
* or agave or maple syrup or a blend of these

Flour blend options: These cookies can be made with a variety of gluten-free flour blends. Equal parts (3/4 cup each) of brown rice flour, GF oat flour and almond meal makes a nice, rich cookie. ¾ cup brown rice flour and 1 ¾ cup oat flour is also quite good. The Oat Rice Baking Mix can be used with great results. Another blend, similar to the Basic Baking Mix includes 1 cup sorghum flour, ¾ cup brown rice flour, ½ cup light buckwheat flour and produces a tender cookie. Press down with a spatula near the end of the baking time if you want "flat" cookies with this option.

Gingersnaps

1 ½ cups teff flour* ¼ cup water
½ cup light buckwheat flour ½ cup oil/butter
2 tsp. baking soda 1/3 cup molasses
½ tsp. sea salt ¼ cup honey**
1 Tbsp. ground ginger 2 tsp. apple cider vinegar
1 tsp. cinnamon 1/2 cup ground flax
¼ tsp. cloves

Combine dry ingredients (left column) in a large mixing bowl. Combine wet ingredients (right column) then mix with dry. Drop by teaspoon onto a baking sheet or stone and bake at 350 degrees for 18-20 minutes. Leave the cookies on the baking sheet for at least 10 minutes after baking before transferring to a cooling rack. **Makes about 4 dozen**
* or sorghum flour. Press flat partway through baking time.
** or agave or maple syrup

Variation: add 1/3 cup carob or cocoa powder plus 2-3 Tbsp. more water for "chocolate snaps".

For really crisp cookies: leave the cookies in the oven at 225 degrees for another 15 minutes or so and then leave them in the oven until the oven is cool. This dries them out nicely. Personally, I like really crisp gingersnaps.

For even "zippier" cookies: add an extra 1 tsp. ground ginger.

Moon Cookies (cookie cutter cookies)

1 ¾ cups GF oat flour

¼ cup light buckwheat flour

¼ cup sorghum flour

Opt: 2 Tbsp. cornmeal

1 tsp. cinnamon

1/8 tsp. ground ginger

1/8 tsp. ground cloves

1 tsp. baking powder

½ tsp. baking soda

½ tsp. sea salt

¼ cup warm water

1/3 cup oil/butter

¼ cup honey*

1 tsp. apple cider vinegar

1/3 cup ground flax

Chocolate version:
   Add 2 Tbsp. molasses
   and 1/3 cup cocoa
   powder. Increase
   honey to 1/3 cup.

Mix dry ingredients (left column) in a mixing bowl. Combine wet ingredients (right column) and then mix thoroughly with dry. Sprinkle counter and dough with sorghum flour. Roll out 1/4 inch thick. Use a round cookie cutter or glass top to cut full moons and crescents from the dough. Bake at 350 degrees for 15-17 minutes, until lightly browned.

* or agave or maple syrup

These cookies were cut into animal shapes when my oldest son was young. With my three new little ones and no cookie cutters in sight, we improvised and cut out round cookies with the top of a small canning jar. Some were full rounds and some were partials where we overlapped a space, so "moon cookies" were born. They love the moon, so these are a real hit with them!

Oat-free Moon Cookies

1 1/3 cup sorghum or teff flour
¼ cup light buckwheat flour
Opt: 2 Tbsp. cornmeal
1 tsp. cinnamon
1/8 tsp. ground ginger
1/8 tsp. ground cloves
1 tsp. baking powder
½ tsp. baking soda
½ tsp. sea salt

½ cup warm water
1/3 cup oil/butter
¼ cup honey*
1 tsp. apple cider vinegar
1/3 cup ground flax
Chocolate version:
   Add 2 Tbsp. molasses
   and 1/3 cup cocoa
   powder. Increase
   honey to 1/3 cup.

Mix dry ingredients (left column) in a mixing bowl. Combine wet ingredients (right column) and then mix thoroughly with dry. Sprinkle counter and dough with sorghum flour. Roll out 1/4 inch thick. Use a round cookie cutter or glass top to cut full moons and crescents from the dough. Place on a baking sheet and bake at 350 degrees for 15-17 minutes, until lightly browned.

* or agave or maple syrup

These make great "staple" cookies as they contain very little oil and sweeteners. They have a nice delicate flavor. My oldest son says they "taste like Christmas".

Scottish Shortbread

1/2 cup oil/butter

2 cup GF oat flour

2/3 cup brown rice flour

1/2 cup honey*

1/4 tsp. sea salt

Either hand-cut butter into the flour or process together in a food processor (the latter is my preference). Add salt and sweetener, and then mix or process until well combined. Press into the bottom of an 8 x 8 baking pan and prick the surface with a fork. Bake at 300 degrees for about 40 minutes (until golden, not browned). Allow to cool for at least ½ hour before cutting.

* or agave or maple syrup. I particularly like them prepared with maple syrup.

It was interesting to find that though shortbread is now most commonly made with white wheat flour, it was traditionally made with oat and even brown rice flour. Neat!

Carob Bars

¼ cup coconut butter
½ cup hot water
½ cup honey
½ cup carob powder
½ cup almond butter

½ cup chopped nuts
3 cups GF rolled oats
¾ cup shredded coconut
½ cup raisins (opt.)
½ tsp. sea salt (opt.)

In a large bowl, whisk together coconut butter, hot water, honey, almond butter and carob powder until smooth (and sea salt, if including). Add remaining ingredients (right column) to this carob mixture and mix well. Pour into an 8 ½ x 11 rectangular baking pan and press down with a spatula. Refrigerate before cutting into bars.

Of all the "carob-trying-to-taste-like-chocolate" recipes out there, I think this is one of the best!

Mint Carob Bars

Prepare Carob Bars as described above except leave out the raisins and add ¾ tsp. of mint extract to the mixture.

Fudge Brownies

15 oz. can black beans   ½ cup cocoa powder
1/3 cup oil/butter   3 Tbsp. light buckwheat flour
2/3 cup honey*   ½ tsp. baking soda
2 tsp. apple cider vinegar   ¼ tsp. sea salt
2 Tbsp. ground flax   opt: ¾ cup chopped nuts

Drain and rinse black beans in a colander. Combine all ingredients in a food processor or blender (except nuts) and blend until smooth. Mix in nuts (if including) then pour into an oiled 9 x 9 baking pan and bake at 350 degrees for 30-35 minutes. Allow to cool before attempting to slice and serve.
* or agave or maple syrup
Opt: For a drier brownie, add less oil or 1-2 Tbsp. more flour.

Your eyes don't fool you. The main ingredient in these brownies is black beans! The beans contribute moistness, fiber and good texture. The brownies are also "grain-free" since the only flour added is from buckwheat, technically not a grain but the seed of an herb.

Carob version: replace cocoa powder with 1 cup carob powder, reduce honey to ½ cup and add 3 Tbsp. each of tahini and molasses, plus 1/3 cup water and another 1/3 cup light buckwheat flour. Presoak ½ cup prunes in hot water, drain and then blend with all ingredients in a blender.

Blender Brownies

¾ cup long grain brown rice

2 tsp. apple cider vinegar

_____

¾-1 cup cocoa powder

½ tsp. baking soda

3 Tbsp. ground flax

opt: 1 cup chopped nuts

2/3 cup water

2/3 cup honey*

opt: 2 Tbsp. molasses

½ cup oil/butter

½ tsp. sea salt

opt: 1/3 cup prunes

  (presoaked)

Soak brown rice in water with vinegar for at least 8 hours (or overnight).   Drain, then process in a blender with the ingredients in the right column.   Pour into a mixing bowl. Using a sieve, sprinkle cocoa powder, ground flax and baking soda into mixture, then whisk together (add nuts, if including).   Pour into an 8 ½ x 11 rectangular baking pan and bake at 350 degrees for about 25 minutes.

* or agave or maple syrup

Carob version: replace cocoa powder with carob powder, reduce honey to ½ cup, plus increase water to ¾ cup, molasses to 1/4 cup, and add 1/4 cup tahini to batter.   It doesn't taste "just like chocolate" but is bliss for those who have to live without!

Rice Pudding

2 cups brown rice

5 ½ cups water

15 oz. can coconut milk

½- ¾ cup raisins

1/3 cup honey

1/8 tsp. sea salt

½ tsp. cinnamon

¼ tsp. nutmeg

Opt: ¼ tsp. ground cardamom

Bring the brown rice and 5 ½ cups water to a boil, then simmer, covered, for about 50 minutes. Add the rest of the ingredients and simmer for at least 20-30 minutes longer, uncovered, stirring frequently. The pudding is done when the rice is quite tender and most of the liquid has been absorbed. Serve warm or chill before serving.

Option: This pudding can also be made with 4 cups of precooked brown rice. In this case, add a cup of water to the other ingredients before simmering for at least 30 minutes.

Sprinkle with nutmeg or cinnamon before serving
for an extra special presentation.

Banana Pudding

1 cup walnuts/pecans/almonds*
1/3 cup dates
Pinch of sea salt

¾ cup water
3/4 cup walnuts
½ cup dates
7 ripe bananas

PREP: Presoak walnuts for at least ½ hour.

Process ingredients in left column in a food processor until finely chopped (holds together when pinched). This is the crust and crumble topping.

Blend water, soaked walnuts and dates (and a pinch of sea salt, if desired) until smooth. Add four of the bananas and blend until smooth again (a pudding-like consistency).

Press three-quarters of the crust into the bottom of a small casserole dish. Thinly slice one banana on top of this crust layer. Pour about one-third of the pudding mixture over top. Slice another banana over this layer. Pour another third of the pudding on top. Slice the last banana on this layer. Top with the rest of pudding. Sprinkle top with remaining crust mixture. Refrigerate briefly before serving.

*any combination of these nuts

It's very important that the bananas you use for this recipe are quite ripe so that the pudding will be nice and sweet.

Option: Add a dash of lemon juice to the banana mixture to reduce browning.

Apple Crisp

3 lb. apples (about 10)
¼ cup oil/butter
¼-1/3 cup maple syrup*
1 ½ cups GF rolled oats

½ cup GF oat flour**
1 tsp. cinnamon
1/8 tsp. sea salt
Opt.: ½ cup walnuts

Peel and slice apples and layer into an 8 ½ x 11 rectangular baking pan. Combine oil/butter and maple syrup in a small saucepan. Heat slightly then mix in the rest of the topping ingredients. Sprinkle topping evenly over apples in pan. Bake at 350 degrees for 35-45 minutes, until golden brown and apples are tender.

* or agave. Honey can also be substituted for the maple syrup, but it browns more quickly, so you'll have to watch the top carefully so it doesn't burn.

** or sorghum, light buckwheat or teff flour

*This dessert is always a hit with company
and at parties and potlucks.*

Blueberry Cobbler

6 cups blueberries

1 cup sorghum flour*

1/3 cup brown rice flour

1/3 cup light buckwheat flour

2 tsp. baking powder

Opt: ½ tsp. cinnamon

1/3 cup honey**

¼ cup oil/butter

1 cup water***

¼ cup ground flax

1 tsp. apple cider vinegar

¼ tsp. sea salt

Place blueberries into the bottom of an 8 ½ x 11 rectangular baking pan. Separately mix dry ingredients (left column) and wet ingredients (right column). Mix lightly together and then pour batter over top of berries. Top with sauce (below).

* or 1 ½ cups GF oat flour

** or agave or maple syrup

*** or non-dairy milk

¼- 1/3 cup honey/maple syrup

3 Tbsp. brown rice flour

½ cup water

Whisk together honey, brown rice flour and water in a small saucepan. Bring almost to a boil and then pour over top of batter. This serves to produce a nice crisp crust and to thicken the berries below. Bake at 350 degrees for 35- 40 minutes.

Peaches, apples, rhubarb and other berries can be substituted for the blueberries. Adjust sweetener and thickener as needed.

Traditional Pie Crust

1 1/3 cups sorghum or teff flour
6 Tbsp. butter
¼- ½ tsp. sea salt
Opt: ¼ cup ground flax

2 Tbsp. maple syrup
1 tsp. apple cider vinegar
3-4 Tbsp. water

Combine all ingredients except for flour and water in a small mixing bowl. Mix flour in until well combined. Add water one tablespoon at a time until mixture begins to hold together well when pinched. Press into a pie plate and bake at 350 degrees for 12-14 minutes. Fill with pie filling (pumpkin filling, apples, etc.) and then bake required amount of time.

An interesting note: *Pie crust is traditionally made with shortening and the meaning of the name of that ingredient has great relevance to the making of a good pie crust. Pie crusts should be light and flaky, and the inclusion of gluten doesn't work to this end. Shortening is added because it "shortens" or cuts the gluten strands in traditional pie crusts made with wheat flour. So preparing a gluten-free pie crust shouldn't be an impossible endeavor, as we are actually trying to "undo" the effect of gluten. The "grittiness" of non-gluten flours, however, doesn't as easily give us the same effect as fine ground wheat flour. I've found sorghum and teff flour work well, yet some might find the dark color of the teff crust unappealing. Both are complementary to pumpkin pie!*

Oat Nut Pie Crust

1 ½ cup GF rolled oats
1 cup pecans or walnuts
¼ tsp. sea salt

3 Tbsp. oil/butter
3 Tbsp. maple syrup*

Process rolled oats and walnuts in food processor until finely chopped. Add rest of ingredients and pulse process until the mixture begins to hold together. Press into a pie plate and bake at 350 degrees for 10-12 minutes. Fill with pie filling (pumpkin filling, apples, etc.) and then bake required amount of time.

* or agave syrup

Pumpkin Pie

1 can pumpkin puree*
½-2/3 cup maple syrup
1 can coconut milk**
1/2 cup brown rice flour***
Opt: 1 Tbsp. molasses

1 tsp. cinnamon
½ tsp. ground ginger
1/8 tsp. nutmeg
1/8 tsp. cloves
½ tsp. sea salt

Whisk together all ingredients in a mixing bowl and then pour into a pie crust- the Oat Nut Pie Crust (pg. 106) or Traditional Pie Crust (pg. 105) work well for this purpose. Sprinkle top with nutmeg. Bake at 350 degrees for 55-60 minutes. Filling will be soft, but will firm up as it cools. Chill and serve.

*15 oz., or about 2 cups mashed pumpkin

** or 1 ½ cup non-dairy milk. Add 1-2 more tablespoons of flour with this alternative.

*** or 2/3 cup sorghum flour. Both flours work great, but sorghum is preferential if the pie is going to be eaten on another day, since it keeps a better texture than the brown rice flour.

Variation: use 2 tsp. pumpkin pie spice in place of the individual spices.

Date Nut Pie Crust *(raw)*

sweet and rich, great for fresh (raw) and frozen pies

1 cup pecans
1 cup walnuts
1 cup dates, pitted

¼+ cup honey (to taste)
¼ - ½ tsp. sea salt (to taste)

Process pecans, walnuts and dates in food processor until well-chopped. Add honey and continue to process until mixture begins to hold together. *Be careful to not over-process.* Press into the bottoms and sides of a pie plate.

Tip: Reserve some of the "dough" to crumble on top of the finished pie.

Date Nut Cookie Balls

Date Nut Pie Crust can be made into cookie balls. Any of the following ingredients can be added to the processor:

> 1 tsp. cinnamon and/or ½ tsp. nutmeg,
> or 1 Tbsp. carob powder,
> or 1-2 Tbsp. orange zest

Roll the dough into balls and serve as is or additionally roll in flaked coconut, ground nuts or carob powder.

As cookies, these make excellent holiday treats and presents.

Fresh Apple Pie (no-bake)

4 Granny Smith apples

2 sweet apples

¼ cup honey

2 tsp. cinnamon

¼ tsp. sea salt

1 tsp. psyllium powder

4 dates, pitted

1 cup raisins

Prepare Date Nut Pie Crust (pg. 108). Press into the bottom and sides of pie plate, reserving a small amount to sprinkle on top of the finished pie.

Peel apples. In food processor, puree three Granny Smith apples and one sweet apple with honey, cinnamon, sea salt, dates and psyllium powder into an applesauce consistency. Allow to sit for a few minutes, then reprocess (to work out any psyllium "lumps"). Pour mixture into a bowl. Mix in raisins. In processor, coarse chop last two apples. Add to bowl mixture. Ideally allow the pie filling to set for about half an hour before pouring into the crust so the raisins have a chance to absorb some of the excess moisture. Pour into crust, smooth top and sprinkle with reserved crust topping. Refrigerate until ready to serve.

Option: Add ½ cup chopped walnuts to pie filling.

Banana Cream Pie *(frozen)*

2 fresh bananas   2/3 cup dates, pitted
4 frozen bananas

Process fresh bananas and dates in a heavy-duty blender (or through a masticating juicer* with the blank in place). Add frozen bananas and process just till well-mixed (want to keep as frozen as possible). Pour into Date Nut Pie Crust (pg. 108) and place in freezer for at least 1-2 hours before serving.
*not a centrifugal juicer

Coconut Banana Cream Pie

2 fresh bananas   2/3 cup dates, pitted
4 frozen bananas   1 cup coconut

Process fresh bananas and dates in a heavy-duty blender (or through a masticating juicer with the blank in place). Add frozen bananas and process just till well-mixed (want to keep as frozen as possible). Mix in coconut (reserve a small amount) and pour into Date Nut Pie Crust (pg. 108). Sprinkle top with the reserved coconut before freezing.
*not a centrifugal juicer

Banana Berry Ice Cream

8-10 frozen bananas
3 cups frozen berries
  (strawberries and/or blueberries)

3/4 cup almonds
  or walnuts

Using the "blank" (not screen) in a masticating juicer*, alternatively process bananas, berries and nuts into a bowl. Stir well. Delicious!
*not a centrifugal juicer

Great topped with fresh berries, chopped nuts, shredded coconut, ground flax and/or chocolate/carob sauce.

For those who can't consume dairy, it's almost worth the purchase of a juicer just to be able to make this tasty and highly nutritious ice cream!

Ice Cream Pie

Press Date Nut Pie Crust (page 108) into a pie plate. Pour Banana Berry Ice Cream (above) or fruit smoothie into the pie shell. Freeze for at least 2 hours. Before serving, remove from freezer and leave at room temperature for 10-15 minutes, or place in refrigerator for about ½ hour. This will allow the pie to soften slightly so it can be cut into slices more easily.

Chocolate Sauce

½ cup honey
¼ cup non-dairy milk
1 Tbsp. oil/butter

3-4 Tbsp. cocoa (to taste)
2 Tbsp. sorghum flour*
pinch of sea salt

Whisk ingredients together in a small saucepan. Simmer until thickened.
* or 1 ½ Tbsp. brown rice flour

Carob Sauce

2 Tbsp. oil/butter
¼-1/3 cup honey*
¼ cup water
3 Tbsp. tahini

2-3 tsp. molasses
1/3 cup carob powder
1 Tbsp. sorghum flour**
¼ tsp. sea salt

Whisk ingredients together in a small saucepan. Simmer until thickened.
* or agave or maple syrup, to taste
** or 2 tsp. brown rice flour

Carob requires less sweetener than cocoa powder.

Information Index

M, N, O, P, Q, R

S, T

U, V, W,X, Y, Z

Recipe Index

A

B

C, D

E, F, G, H, I, J, K

L, M, N

O, P

Other cookbooks in Kim Wilson's
Everyday Wholesome Eating series
are also packed full of simple and tasty
gluten-free and allergen-free recipes.
Round out your mealtime needs with more recipes for
wholesome soups, salads, entrees, snacks, desserts, etc.

Everyday Wholesome Eating - a whole foods plant-based cookbook, featuring over 150 simple and tasty recipes as well as extensive information to help with the transition to a natural diet.   **145 gluten-free recipes!**

Everyday Wholesome Eating. . . In The Raw - an all-raw recipe book featuring over 200 simple and tasty dishes as well as a thorough introduction to raw foods and the preparation of such.   **200 gluten-free recipes!**

My Soup Book - fifty wholesome and hearty soups and soup accompaniments.   **47 gluten-free recipes!**
(Soon to be expanded into "**Everyday Soup** - 52 seasonal and all-season soups, stews and chowders plus accompaniments").

For other books in the "Everyday Wholesome Eating"
series, visit **www.simplynaturalhealth.com**